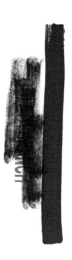

SAVING GOTHAM

ALSO BY TOM FARLEY, MD

Prescription for a Healthy Nation
(with Deborah A. Cohen)

SAVING GOTHAM

A Billionaire Mayor, Activist

Doctors, and the Fight for

Eight Million Lives

TOM FARLEY, MD

W. W. Norton & Company
Independent Publishers Since 1923
New York • London

For information about permission to reproduce selections from this book,
write to Permissions, W. W. Norton & Company, Inc.,
500 Fifth Avenue, New York, NY 10110

For information about special discounts for bulk purchases,
please contact W. W. Norton Special Sales
at specialsales@wwnorton.com or 800-233-4830

Manufacturing by Quad Graphics
Book design by Dana Sloan
Production manager: Louise Mattarelliano

ISBN: 978-0-393-07124-5

W. W. Norton & Company, Inc.
500 Fifth Avenue, New York, N.Y. 10110
www.wwnorton.com

W. W. Norton & Company Ltd.
Castle House, 75/76 Wells Street, London W1T 3QT

1 2 3 4 5 6 7 8 9 0

To Alice, who enables my eccentricities,
and Emily, Joanna, Helen, and Rebecca,
of whom I am very proud

Contents

SAVING GOTHAM

Preface

In June 2006 I flew to Atlanta to give a talk at a conference on public health law. The attendees were mostly lawyers, professors, and officials from state health departments and the Centers for Disease Control and Prevention (CDC)—a rumpled, polite, and long-winded group that debated topics like government-mandated vaccination registries. But the keynote talk was to be delivered by Michael Bloomberg, then in his second term as mayor of New York City. At the packed closing session, Bloomberg strutted into the conference hall wearing a Wall Street suit, surrounded by a pack of large men wearing coiled security earphones. Trailing him was a compact, boyish, but intense-looking man with a bounce in his step whom I recognized as Tom Frieden, the city's health commissioner.

At the time I was a professor of public health in New Orleans. I had worked for the CDC and for the state health department in Louisiana, where I had learned to be contemptuous of politicians. None of them understood anything about health except that people demanded medical care regardless of the cost; the Democrats wanted to give people more of that care and the Republicans wanted to cut government spending on it. I knew little about Bloomberg except that he was a Wall Street tech billionaire who had banned smoking in bars. I slouched in the back, not expecting much.

1

But when Bloomberg began talking, reading his speech at ticker-tape pace in his Boston accent, I straightened up in my chair. He spoke about smoking as the nation's biggest enemy. About getting illegal guns off the street. About why the city was distributing its own brand of condoms and giving sterile needles to drug users. Public health people talked like that, but a mayor? "We rely on the forceful application of law—democratically debated and approved—as the principal instrument of public health policy," he said. These ideas were political losers. This guy was very, very different.

Tom Frieden sat in the front row holding a binder in his lap, hanging on his boss's words. He had a reputation for being smart and pushy. Though I had never met him, I knew that he had gone through the same training program at the CDC that I had. It hit me that Frieden was behind the ideas in Bloomberg's speech. A smart, powerful politician was actually listening to a man with life-saving but politically dangerous ideas. The two were a combination I thought I'd never see.

Those of us who work in public health fight diseases in entire populations rather than one person at a time. Rather than treat sickness, we prevent it by acting "upstream." If the tools of medical care are drugs and surgery, the tools of public health are information, policies, and laws. Doctors treat cholera victims with intravenous fluids, but public health people prevent cholera by mandating clean water and sewage systems.

A year earlier, a colleague and I had published a book arguing that, just as we had beaten cholera, we could beat the leading killers of our time with public health actions. Nearly four in ten people in America died from chronic diseases like heart disease, cancer, and diabetes. People could avoid those diseases by behaving in a healthier way, particularly avoiding smoking, eating healthier food, and being physically active. But most people can't behave that way consistently because they are preoccupied and stressed and living in world that, day after day, makes it easy to do what is unhealthy and difficult to do the opposite. If we want to be healthy as a nation, my colleague and I wrote, we should change our everyday world to make healthy behaviors easier. Now Bloomberg was saying the same thing. He told the conference, "Public health succeeds by making the healthy choice the default social option."

Every important action taken in public health incites opposition, because it means changing society. And that often makes the work of public health heartbreaking. Those of us who do it see people suffering and dying from preventable diseases, and we dream of taking simple actions to fix the causes. And then, because we face strong political headwinds, we often end up running insignificant pilot programs or writing proposals that are ignored. On the plane home from Atlanta, I couldn't stop thinking about the combination of Bloomberg and Frieden. This looked like a once-in-a-century aligning of forces, a chance to do something big.

Two weeks later I e-mailed Frieden to ask if I could work for him at the New York City Department of Health and Mental Hygiene. He invited me to come to New York to talk, and a few months later I began a year as his adviser.

I wasn't disappointed. Frieden indeed had huge ambitions, and he was leading a band of activist doctors on a mission to save the life of every New Yorker. He also had Mayor Bloomberg's ear. As Frieden and his true believers changed the focus of the health department to modern health problems, they were transforming that agency and redefining public health. I joined the club and advised him on subjects as wide-ranging as drug overdoses and salt levels in food. It was a thrilling time. But Bloomberg's second term was drawing to a close, so at the end of the year I returned to my job as a professor.

Afterward I began writing a book about the New York City health department. In late 2008 and early 2009, I interviewed Tom Frieden and two dozen of his staff for the book. Then things changed. President Barack Obama asked Frieden to be the director of the CDC; the New York City Council revised a law so that Bloomberg could run for a third term; and Bloomberg asked me to succeed Frieden as health commissioner. So in the spring of 2009 I put the book aside and moved to New York City.

During the Bloomberg years, the city health department attacked what we saw as America's biggest killer—smoking. It then went after heart disease, stroke, hypertension, and obesity by mounting assaults on trans fats, salt in processed food, and sugary drinks. None of these initiatives happened easily. They took place only after painstaking—often repeated and circular—review and skirmishing within the health department, followed by wrangling within City Hall. Many ideas died in the process. Others made it into the sunlight, only to be killed by the state or federal government or by the courts. Still others survived and thrived.

In the early 1990s Al Sommer, then dean of the School of Public Health at Johns Hopkins University, approached businessman Michael Bloomberg for a donation for his school. In their first conversation, Sommer compared public health to medicine, hitting hard on the idea that public health actions save lives wholesale instead of retail. "Mike got it like that," Sommer said to me, snapping his fingers. Later a Johns Hopkins administrator said to Sommer, "I don't know what you told Mike Bloomberg, but he's going around telling everybody that the School of Public Health saves more lives than the medical school will in its entire history." Sommer and Bloomberg, who later became friends, liked the phrase. Over the years, they played with it and made it into a slogan that Sommer trademarked for what is now the Johns Hopkins Bloomberg School of Public Health: *Protecting health, saving lives—millions at a time.*

This book tells the story of what happened when a group of dedicated people tried in the nation's largest city to make that slogan real—to save lives, millions at a time.

PART ONE

1

"Things are going to get really exciting."

Near midnight Chris Gallin was at home at his desk, paying bills, when he felt his left shoulder and arm getting stiff. He had smoked his last ciga- rette of the day an hour earlier. In his job managing a family construction business, he didn't lift or carry things, but he thought he might have pulled a muscle somehow. Then his shoulder started to hurt. He tried moving it, but that didn't help. He wondered if it was heartburn, so he tried an antacid, but the pain only grew worse. And that's when he knew. He walked to his bedroom and told to his wife to call 911, because he was having a heart attack.

At the hospital, the doctors told Gallin and his wife that he had a com- plete blockage of the artery that supplies the main part of the heart. They called it "the widow-maker." They were surprised that he had made it to the hospital. He was forty-six years old.

• • •

At eight a.m. on January 22, 2002, Tom Frieden climbed the steps from the number six subway into a small triangular park in lower Manhattan, lugging a roll-on suitcase that held a stack of papers and his laptop. He had flown in from India at ten o'clock the night before and had slept a few hours at a friend's apartment. He paused, looked across the park at a

7

ten-story building—the headquarters of the Department of Health and
Mental Hygiene—and thought: *This is it.*

The gray building is graced with art deco touches from the 1930s. The
exterior walls feature octagonal silver medallions with muscular Greek-
looking figures washing themselves or grinding medicine with mortar
and pestle. Nearer the top, chiseled in stone on all four sides, are the last
names of twenty-six heroes in health. There is Jenner, who invented vaccination to tame smallpox, and Lind, who eradicated scurvy with lem-
ons. There is Semmelweis, who discovered that deadly infections were
being spread by doctors in hospitals, and Nightingale, who showed how
to prevent those infections. And Koch, who discovered the bacteria that
cause many diseases, and Ehrlich, who produced the first antibiotics to
kill them.

In 2002 the building headquartered two departments, the Department
of Health and the Department of Mental Health, Mental Retardation, and
Alcoholism Services. The two answered to one commissioner—as of that
day, Frieden. The combined agency, with some 6,000 staff and a budget of
$1.6 billion, was a conglomerate. The health department tested the city's
drinking water, inspected restaurants, enforced vaccination requirements
for children, repaired peeling lead-based paint that poisoned toddlers, and
traced contacts to control the spread of tuberculosis and sexually trans-
mitted diseases. It issued millions of birth and death certificates and used
the data to calculate health statistics. It supplied nurses to more than one
thousand schools and inspected tens of thousands of day care centers.
Its mental hygiene arm funded treatment for alcoholism, drug addiction,
mental illness, and developmental delay. What the health department
didn't do was provide basic medical care. That was the job of private doctors, federally funded community health centers, and the city's Health
and Hospitals Corporation. In fact, the city health department had little
involvement with the medical care system.

The city had established the health department nearly two hundred
years earlier as a committee to battle epidemics of infectious diseases.
Since then the agency had grown fitfully as it took on new jobs—from
administering polio vaccinations to establishing methadone clinics—in

response to subsequent crises. But like most health departments in the year 2002, New York City's did very little to combat the city's biggest killers: heart disease, stroke, cancer, and diabetes.

. . .

When I first met Tom Frieden, I was struck by his youthful looks and his frenetic energy, which gave him the look of a twelve-year-old boy playing commissioner. He seemed to speak twice as fast as the hyper New Yorkers around him. Listening to him was like watching a game of pinball, as he ricocheted among numbers, biology, history, anecdotes, and local politics. He kept two folded-up three-by-five index cards in his shirt pocket, and he would often stop abruptly in midsentence, pull them out, and make cryptic notes in five-point font. Then he'd refold the cards, slide them back in his pocket, and start racing again, usually on a different topic. He quoted obscure scientific papers and the sayings of political rogues. Running over statistics, he sounded like a combination of a science professor gushing about his experiments and a beat reporter rattling off the details of a juicy scandal, describing numbers with words like *fascinating* and *extraordinary*. His intensity was fierce but also joyous; he often interrupted himself with rapid-fire one-liners, laughing with his entire torso.

When I arrived at the health department in 2007, Frieden briefed me as only he could, streaming ideas that were both detailed and grandiose. His antitobacco program wanted to slash the number of stores selling cigarettes, but he couldn't figure out how to do it legally and politically. He was creating a $27 million electronic medical record system and installing it in a thousand doctors' offices. He was writing an opinion piece for the *Journal of the American Medical Association* on how to restructure the $2 trillion U.S. health care system, but he didn't have time to finish it, so could I help? Then he took a call from a labor leader who had built his own health care system for his union members, which was second to none. "We need to learn from that guy," Frieden said. The New York State Restaurant Association was suing him over the department's requirement that restaurants post calorie counts on their menu boards. When the health department did a first-ever citywide examination survey of New Yorkers, they found sky-high levels of mercury in the Chinese, who Frieden suspected were acquiring the metal from fish caught in polluted waters. To get more new mothers to breastfeed, he was pushing every public hospital to banish giveaways of infant formula. New Yorkers were losing their hearing—maybe because of the screeching subways—and he wanted to figure out how to fix the trains because the MTA wouldn't. There was so much more, but he had to get back to his e-mail.

Those index cards with daily to-do lists were a habit Frieden had picked up years earlier as a medical resident. He divided each card, always folded exactly in half, into tiny sections—people to call, papers to read, e-mails to send. If at the end of the day he wasn't able to cross an item off his list, he had to rewrite it on the next day's card—a personal failure for which, according to an assistant, "he could not be consoled." Frieden also kept weekly to-do lists, which he numbered for each week on the job in New York. And he kept monthly to-do lists. And yearly to-do lists.

Frieden suffered from a burden of urgency that was almost painful to watch. People were dying from preventable causes in New York City, and he took every death personally. It was as if a Code Blue were called every day and only he could run over, slap on the paddles, and shock the victim back to life. He walked so fast that people had to break into a trot to keep pace. When he asked people questions, he often interrupted their answers after the first few words because knew where they were going. When answering e-mails, his response was often one letter only—Y or N. "Have you seen him eat?" one of his assistants said to me. "He doesn't chew!" And sure enough, one day when we met for lunch, I noticed that he dropped his head and seemed to vacuum the food in one long slurp.

• • •

Tom Frieden grew up in New York City's suburbs, the son of a cardiologist in solo practice who took calls from his patients every night but also aspired to be a scholar, reading medical journals voraciously. Frieden idolized his father, who raised Tom on medicine and politics. "You gotta help the people," the father told the son.

During the summers between his terms in medical school, Tom Frieden traveled to Nicaragua. The country had just seen the Sandinista revolution overthrow the Somoza dictatorship. In the 1980s the revolutionary movements in Central America became a kind of siren call to American leftists, especially in health. The Sandinistas were copying Cuba, which, despite its poverty, had higher immunization rates than did New York City. "The Sandinistas early on were very inspiring," Frieden told me. They "had very good health campaigns. Vaccination, oral rehydration. They did clinic building. They did maternal mortality stuff." He began working with a New York City–based organization called the National Central America Health Rights Network, creating a newsletter on Central America that he edited for ten years. While working on Central American issues, he dealt with a tall young man named Bill de Blasio, who would later become mayor of New York City. As the years went by, Frieden grew disenchanted with the Sandinistas: "They became very corrupt."

After he finished his medical training, he joined the Epidemic Intelligence Service (EIS), a two-year program run by the Centers for Disease Control and Prevention (CDC) to turn doctors into disease detectives. The CDC farmed out many of its EIS officers to state and local health departments for training. Frieden angled for and landed the spot in New York City, where he investigated an astonishing twenty-four disease outbreaks in two years.

One of those outbreaks erupted into a national crisis: the epidemic of drug-resistant tuberculosis in people with AIDS, spread mainly within hospitals. Experts around the country—including me—saw the epidemic in nearly apocalyptic terms: it was a sign that AIDS, by making hundreds of thousands of people susceptible to infections, was transforming tuberculosis into an uncontrollable problem. So after his training ended, Frieden took charge of the city's tuberculosis program to control it.

The solution to the crisis, as he saw it, was not a cure for AIDS, which was at best many years away. The solution was just to make sure—really, really sure—that people with TB took their medicines until they were cured so that they didn't spread the infection to others. That meant, more than anything, assigning health department workers to watch TB patients swallow every single one of their pills, either at home or in the clinic. That simple process earned the bureaucratic name directly observed therapy (DOT). It had worked in the world's most destitute countries. Why not New York City?

As Frieden threw his energy into the TB program, he got some management advice from an old hand. "You may work twice as many hours and three times as fast as others," the man told him, "but that's still only six people. And what six people do in a large organization is irrelevant." So Frieden leveraged the panic over the outbreak into millions in additional funding from both the city and the CDC, with which he expanded the TB program's staff from 200 to 830. Now he had the army to apply DOT to the thousands of New Yorkers with tuberculosis.

One day he gave a tour to a visiting TB expert from overseas, proudly displaying the data he used to track his program. The expert asked Frieden "the single question that changed my life," as he later called it: "You diagnosed 3,811 patients last year. How many of them did you cure?"

"And I didn't know!" Frieden told me. "And I was tremendously humiliated." For all his numbers, he lacked the one that mattered the most. From that point on, he instituted "cohort reviews" of each individual patient and tracked cure rates religiously. The bigger lesson was: measure the outcome.

Frieden's program worked stunningly well. The 3,811 cases of tuberculosis that were diagnosed the year he took over the program was the highest number on record. Five years later the case count had shrunk to 1,600, and it would soon hit historic lows.

In 1997 the director for tuberculosis control for the World Health Organization asked Frieden to help manage India's massive TB program. "I got there, and I was at the top of my game," he told me. "I had written in the *New England Journal of Medicine*, the *Lancet*, and everywhere else. I was well known and lauded in the U.S." During a year of bureaucratic hiring delays, he traveled intermittently to India, reviewed the nation's program, and sent instructions to Indian public health officials. They ignored him. They hadn't heard of him, didn't care what he had done in

New York City, and believed anything done in New York wouldn't apply
to their country anyway.

Later, after living in India for a while, Frieden realized they were
right: "In fact, I *didn't* know the vast majority of what I needed to know
about TB in India." So he began traveling extensively around the country, listening to frontline TB program staff. "Within a year, I knew more
about what was happening in the field than anyone else," he said. He
tried to gain Indians' respect through sheer relentlessness, volunteering
for any task that came in his direction. "I'm a mule for work," he told me.
He wrote later, "Every day for the first two years I was [in India], I would
leave the office, often at 9 or 10 o'clock at night, and ask myself, '1,000
people died from TB in India today, and what the hell did I do about it!?'"

A colleague who traveled to India years later found the Indian health
officials in awe of Frieden. "*Nobody* works harder than Dr. Tom," they
told her. Five years after he arrived, the Indian TB program had trained
200,000 staff and increased the percent of people with TB treated with
DOT from near zero to over 50 percent, which amounted to more than
600,000 patients. Frieden needed to estimate how many lives his work
would save. He figured that, as of 2002, the TB program in India would
save 200,000 lives. To keep a tally after he left, he had the program set up
a running "lives saved" counter on its website.

In the fall of 2001, as New York City and the rest of the nation grieved
over the 9/11 attacks and trembled over the anthrax scare that followed,
Tom Frieden wanted to come home. He spotted an opportunity with the
upcoming city election. Rudy Giuliani was ending his term as mayor, and
the Democrat who won the primary was Mark Green, the city's public advocate. In the general election, Green faced an unlikely Republican
candidate, a tech-and-media billionaire and political newcomer named
Michael Bloomberg. Green was so confident that he would win that
before the election his staff contacted Frieden about serving as his future
health commissioner. Green's election looked guaranteed right up to the
day Bloomberg beat him.

The world now knows Michael Bloomberg, the confident and sometimes caustic mayor, but he started his campaign as an unknown. The

father of the data terminals that were essential for Wall Street traders, Bloomberg paraded his $4 billion fortune as a political asset, saying in a campaign ad, "I won't ask special interests for a dime." He played up his differentness: "I don't do the conventional." The press wasn't sure what to make of him, but he kept them entertained. He was a talker, mostly about himself, who kept his aides vigilant by saying whatever he thought. In this heavily Democratic city, he called school prayer "an excellent idea. . . . It is the way I grew up and I didn't turn out so bad."

And when asked about health, the other candidates stayed on safe ground by promising to get poor children health insurance, but Bloomberg blazed his own trail. "There's an enormous number of people who come down with illnesses that could be prevented through education," he said. "Diabetes, coming through diet, abuse of the diet; asthma, dirty air, and not knowing how to clean; substance abuse; smoking-related illnesses . . . somebody has to focus on those." Preventing diseases through education? It was so far from ordinary campaign-speak that *The New York Times* treated it as a gaffe.

After his surprise victory, Bloomberg had to choose heads for more than forty city agencies. Because he had financed his own campaign, he didn't have to repay favors with political appointments. He had a formal transition committee, but for informal advice on a health commissioner, he turned to his friend from Johns Hopkins, Al Sommer. After the committee turned up Frieden's name, Sommer remembers getting phone calls from people he hadn't spoken to for a long time, calling just to say hello and incidentally mentioning that Frieden, whom they happened to know, would make a terrific health commissioner.

Back in India, Frieden began plotting a health strategy for New York City. He started by downloading the fifty-page book of statistics published annually by the health department. In the year 2000, the city had just over eight million inhabitants. They were grouped in five boroughs, each of which was crowded enough to qualify as a city in its own right: Manhattan (the borough most visitors think of as New York City) with 1.5 million people, Brooklyn with 2.5 million, Queens with 2.2 million, the Bronx with 1.5 million, and often-overlooked Staten Island with 440,000. The city had no majority race or ethnic group. The largest group, non-Hispanic whites, made up just 35 percent of the population, Hispanics followed at 27 percent, and non-Hispanic blacks at 24 percent. More than a third of New Yorkers were immigrants, and over half of the babies born in the city were to immigrant mothers.

Of the eight million New Yorkers that year, 60,839 had died. The ways they died reflected the twentieth century's revolution in health. In 1900 the leading killers had been tuberculosis and pneumonia; heart disease and cancer had been relatively infrequent causes of death. By 2000, tuberculosis was rare and pneumonia an uncommon killer, but 24,768 of the deaths—or over 40 percent—were caused by heart disease. Another 14,100, nearly a quarter, were due to cancer.

Smoking was behind many of those deaths. To estimate how many, Frieden did a back-of-the-envelope calculation, assigning rough percentages of deaths attributable to smoking for each cause—for example, 30 percent of heart attacks, 90 percent of lung cancers, 30 percent of other cancers, and 50 percent of strokes. He quickly concluded that roughly 20 percent of all the city's deaths were caused by smoking. Like everyone else in public health, he had known that smoking was a big killer, but the size of the problem shocked him. For the previous ten years he had been immersed in tuberculosis: "I thought, wow, they haven't controlled smoking yet?" He decided then that if he got the New York City job, smoking would be his top enemy.

Frieden remembers getting an e-mail from Sommer asking if he wanted to be considered for health commissioner. He wrote back that his taking the job "would only make sense if he [Bloomberg] is willing to take on tobacco, and that's very political. . . . It wasn't a condition, I just didn't want to waste everyone's time."

Sommer remembers the exchange differently. It was over the telephone, and Sommer casually asked Frieden what health problems he would tackle if he got the job. Smoking, Frieden said emphatically. Sommer was incredulous. The World Trade Center site was still smoldering, and the anthrax-laced letter mystery remained unsolved. "Tom, ever hear of nine-eleven?" he asked. "Ever hear of bioterrorism?" Sommer said Frieden told him, yes, of course he'd deal with bioterrorism too, but smoking would kill far more people.

Frieden flew to the United States to interview. Sommer must have tipped off Bloomberg, because according to Frieden, the mayor—a former smoker—spent the first twelve minutes of the interview all but ignoring him and haranguing his deputy mayor of operations, Mark Shaw—who still enjoyed cigars—about smoking. Do you know what a huge problem smoking is? he said. It would be like three jumbo jetliners crashing into a mountain every day. It's the biggest public health problem of our time. We've just got to do something about it.

When Bloomberg finally got around to talking to Frieden, as the mayor's chief of staff Peter Madonia put it, "I don't think it was five minutes into the conversation that it was clear to me there was a complete mind-meld between Mike and Tom."

When I first met Frieden, he had on his bookshelf a framed picture of Bloomberg shaking his hand. Taped to it was a piece of paper with the words that the mayor had said to Frieden and his other new commissioners: "It's your agency. Don't screw it up."

. . .

When Frieden arrived in January 2002, the New York City health department was, in the damning words of one employee, "a standard government agency." It was "process-oriented instead of outcome-oriented." Under former mayor Giuliani, its job had been less to promote health than to respond to complaints. Other employees were much harsher about the agency culture. The workers "punched a clock. They didn't collaborate. They hid data that made them look bad." The city's practicing doctors, if they knew anything about the department, thought it "a sleepy, backwater place that would probably never change." Within the two weeks of my own arrival at the department in 2007, I met two people who had quit in frustration in the late 1990s and then rejoined after Frieden took over.

Donna Shelley, a physician, had joined the department in 1999 to run a new tobacco control program. At that time, money had come to the agency from the "Master Settlement Agreement" between state attorneys general and the tobacco companies over Medicaid costs. Shelley, impatient and demanding, fumed at what she saw as the lazy atmosphere. When she asked one of her employees to meet with her at 4:55, he would look at his watch and say, "Well, I'm leaving in five minutes." "Ninety percent of the people there deserved to be fired," she told me. "It was impossible to get anything done. I was bumping heads with everybody all the time." One day a senior department official called her into his office and told her to back off. She was upsetting too many people.

Even before he came to New York, Tom Frieden made it clear that he would run a different kind of department. From India, he sent e-mails to high-level department staff, demanding reams of data about their programs: what did they do, why did they do it, what population were they trying to reach, who did they actually reach, and how did they know if they were successful? The e-mails "sent shock waves through the agency," an assistant in the commissioner's office recalled. "People had never been asked this kind of question. . . . They had no idea what their population . . . served was. They didn't have numerators, they didn't have denominators, they didn't even *think* in numerators and denominators. . . . I think people started to quake."

The new health commissioner wouldn't waste his time with "process"—about who did what. Shortly after he arrived, the agency staff briefed Frieden about one unit that was disorganized enough to be in trouble with a federal regulatory agency. "It was a mess managerially," he told me. "It was *bad*." A staff member in the commissioner's office proposed a solution: hire a consultant to do a "process analysis," then set up a Continuing Quality Improvement program. Frieden had an entirely different take. The problem with the unit was the man running it, who had kept all the files himself and then couldn't keep track of them. So Frieden fired him.

He wanted numbers that measured what mattered. Just as he returned to New York City, Frieden had visited his father, who was now in a nursing home, dying. He described the visit in a talk at a health conference. "And in the very last conversation I ever had with him, before he faded,

I said 'Dad, I'm going to be health commissioner for New York City.' He was happy to hear that. I said, 'Dad, I want to be the best health commissioner.' And he said, in the last words he ever spoke to me, 'How would you know?'" It was why Tom Frieden saw his job as saving as many lives as he could. And why he had to count them.

But Frieden was more than just "outcome-oriented." He was, in Donna Shelley's words, "incapable of process." He wasn't deliberately rude; he was just too impatient to be polite or to explain himself. He would demand, decide, and act, without communicating with the people he needed to carry out his orders. Shelley remembers an early meeting in his office with officials from the American Cancer Society. Ten minutes into the meeting Frieden, apparently feeling the conversation wasn't worth his time, just stood up from the head of the conference table, walked to his desk, and started working on some papers. Shelley said later, "I looked at these people and I thought, 'Oh my god, this is so rude!'" Sure, the meeting was going nowhere, but "we all learn early on as children that we have to engage in some kind of process with people." She thought, "I don't know anybody who acts like that."

• • •

By taking on smoking, Tom Frieden had certainly chosen the right target. He soon refined his initial back-of-the-envelope estimate of the number of New Yorkers killed by smoking to "more than 12,000 adults a year"— more than AIDS, alcohol, suicide, and homicide combined. Half of these smoking-related deaths happened in people under sixty-five. Chris Gallin, who survived his heart attack, was nearly one of them. And people who died from smoking didn't just drop dead—they suffered and lingered from it, paralyzed by stroke, breathless from emphysema, or in pain from cancer. The medical costs associated with smoking ran to more than $4 billion a year in New York City alone—costs that everyone ended up paying through taxes and health insurance premiums.

Coming in, Commissioner Frieden made sure that everyone, both inside and outside the health department, knew exactly how determined he was to combat smoking. "For the last ten-plus years, my enemy was the tuberculosis bacteria," he told reporters in his first press interviews, "but now my enemy is a really low-life form, tobacco executives."

But what exactly was Frieden going to do? People's reasons for smoking defied all logic. Nearly forty years after the first surgeon general's report, everyone—*everyone*—knew that it could kill you, yet one in five adults in New York City still smoked. Every year the small fraction who quit or died were replaced by teenagers taking their first puffs. Kids tried cigarettes to look grown-up and cool and became hooked before they knew it, then struggled to break the habit the rest of their lives. In the decade before Frieden arrived, smoking rates in New York City had not budged.

Before the new health commissioner could figure out his antismoking strategy, Mayor Bloomberg began his. In Frieden's third week on the job, the mayor announced his budget for the year. To fill a $4.8 billion budget gap opened by the city's post-9/11 economic slowdown, he proposed to cut funding for most city agencies, including shrinking the police force and closing care centers for the elderly, in addition to raising some fees and taxes. A key piece of the budget package was a leap in the city's cigarette tax from 8 cents to $1.50, which would make it the nation's highest and raise the price of a pack from a little more than $5.00 to nearly $7.00. The city needed the money, but Bloomberg was sold on the health benefit, telling reporters, "The numbers are clear, you raise taxes, the kids smoke less."

Bloomberg was right. Economists had repeatedly shown that even though tobacco was an addictive drug, when the price went up, people bought fewer cigarettes, smoked less, and quit more. Later Frieden, playing catch-up, used these studies to estimate that Bloomberg's $1.42 tax increase would cut smoking rates in teens by 15 percent and prompt 70,000 adult smokers to quit.

In the health department, Donna Shelley had her own plan to combat smoking. In the years before Frieden arrived, she had visited the top tobacco control programs in the country and consulted experts. She favored a tax increase, among other ideas. She wanted to testify in favor of a cigarette tax, but Giuliani's people had muzzled her. With the best ideas forbidden, she was paying nonprofits to organize teenagers against smoking, under the label "youth empowerment." When she first saw the energy and political power that Frieden and Bloomberg brought to smoking, she was in awe. "Oh my god, this is going to get easy," she thought. But instead, she quickly found herself frustrated. Frieden wasn't about to follow her strategy. He had his own ideas. Among them, he wanted to treat smoking as he had treated TB.

The analogy was this: think of smoking as a disease. Among smokers who weren't "cured," that disease was fatal about one-third of the time. But the disease was treatable. If doctors spent as little as five or ten minutes counseling their patients to quit smoking, Frieden gleaned from research papers, the patients were 50 percent more likely to quit. Giving smokers nicotine patches, nicotine gum, or other medications increased the quit rate even more. Smokers visited doctors often, but their doctors did a terrible job of treating smoking, asking only about two-thirds of them about their habit, counseling only about one-fifth of them to quit, and treating only 2 percent of them with medications.

Frieden put some numbers into a spreadsheet and did another quick estimate. Close to 200,000 of the city's million-odd smokers "could quit with better care," he figured, and if they did, it could save nearly 60,000 lives. All he needed to do, then, was get New York City's doctors to ask every single patient if he or she smoked and to provide counseling to all the smokers who wanted to quit.

The idea was more than ambitious. Shelley thought it delusional. To most doctors, counseling patients to quit smoking was a waste of precious time. And even if counseling increased quitting by from 4 to 6 percent, the result would still be a 94 percent failure rate. And the health department had little leverage over doctors anyway.

Frieden wasn't deterred. After all, if the Indian medical system could treat a million people for tuberculosis, why couldn't the New York City medical system treat a million people for smoking?

He tried to provoke doctors into thinking differently by writing a newsletter to them. At the bottom of the first page he wrote in boldface, "Failure to provide optimal counseling and treatment is failure to meet the standard of care—and could be considered malpractice!"

The state medical society was incensed. "That cannot possibly be what our city health policy is," its lawyer told the *New York Post*. Some doctors responded with angry letters and phone calls. Their patients were dealing with lots of health problems, the doctors said, and they were doing the best they could to address them all. Besides, doctors weren't being paid to counsel smokers.

As Frieden probed for ideas, Donna Shelley had more conflicts with him. "He started with some very weird policy ideas that were not mainstream," she said. But mostly, she was frustrated by his style of demanding information and making decisions without telling her what he was doing, let alone listening to her advice. After her earlier fights in the department she had considered leaving the agency, and now she quit.

· · ·

Gracie Mansion is a Victorian house set in a grassy wooded park overlooking the Hudson, an island of space and tranquility in blaring Manhattan. It is traditionally the mayor's residence, but Bloomberg passed over it in favor of his Upper East Side townhouse. In May 2002, Tom Frieden hosted a round table meeting at Gracie, with smoking experts from universities, advocacy organizations, and health departments in Massachusetts and California. The location told everyone that the meeting was important and that Frieden had the support of the mayor.

During the months before the round table, Frieden read voraciously about smoking prevention and tested his evolving ideas on various experts, from mainstream thinkers to those on the fringe. Although he said the purpose of the Gracie meeting was to get others' opinions, by the time he held it, he already had a detailed slide deck on smoking in New York City and what he proposed to do about it.

His proposal had five pieces: taxation, legal action, education, cessation, and evaluation. He celebrated Mayor Bloomberg's tobacco tax proposal, which was coming up for a vote soon, mentioned expanding the indoor smoking ban to "all workplaces," said the city might "pursue litigation" against the tobacco companies, suggested he would "educate providers on cessation options," and promised to track smoking rates with an annual telephone survey.

The experts told Frieden that coaxing doctors to do a better job treating their smoking patients would be an uphill slog. It wasn't just because of doctors' "colossal ignorance" but also because the insurance plans didn't pay them for it. The Massachusetts people touted their tough antismoking television ads. The Californians promoted their new state law prohibiting smoking in bars and restaurants. The group warned Frieden to avoid taking "over the top" steps like banning smoking outdoors in parks.

The health commissioner took one thing from the meeting: "What really came out was smoke-free [policies]. That smoke-free was a wedge issue. You would change social norms, you would get smokers to quit, and you protect nonsmokers."

Of course, indoor smoking bans protect nonsmokers from getting lung cancer from secondhand smoke, but they have also had surprising spinoff benefits. In the 1990s, when some hospitals and other employers banned smoking indoors, researchers noticed that smokers weren't just going outside to smoke. Many were quitting. And nonsmoking employees were deciding that if secondhand smoke was dangerous at work, they didn't want smokers around them anywhere else. The rules started to make smoking socially unacceptable, which appeared to be driving down smoking rates overall.

The experts left the round table excited that the mayor of New York and his new health commissioner were joining the fight against tobacco. Donna Shelley, who joined the meeting as an outside expert, was stunned at how, after his early oddball ideas, Frieden now grasped the state of the science. "I remember really admiring him," she said later. "I remember feeling like maybe I shouldn't have left. Things are going to get really exciting."

By the end of the meeting, Frieden had a plan that he hoped would save the lives of tens of thousands of New Yorkers. And he knew what dragon he would slay first. He was going to pass a law banning smoking in some 13,000 bars and restaurants, all of whose managers would hate it.

2

"I need a one-pager on lives saved."

Tom Frieden ended many of his lectures with a quote from Dr. Hermann Biggs, a medical officer in the late 1800s and early 1900s who pleaded for New York City to invest in prevention: "Public health is purchasable. Within natural limitations, a community can determine its own death rate." For over twenty years, Biggs led the health department through its high point in battling infectious diseases. He founded the city's bacteriology laboratory and was one of the first to test for the bacteria that cause tuberculosis and cholera. He stopped an epidemic of typhus by quarantining immigrants arriving with the disease. In 1897 he persuaded the Board of Health, over fierce resistance by the city's physicians, to require doctors to report the names of their patients with tuberculosis to the health department. That act enabled Frieden to control tuberculosis almost a century later.

In the 1800s cities were hives of contagion. In those early days of the industrial revolution, people for the first time crowded near factories, packing filthy tenements without plumbing or waste disposal. The lack of running water spread dysentery and cholera, and the poor ventilation spread tuberculosis. Epidemics of yellow fever cropped up as mosquitos thrived in newly cleared, swampy land close to humans.

To prevent those diseases, the city needed to issue orders, particularly for quarantine and sanitation. It was yellow fever that prompted New York City's Common Council in 1805 to establish a Board of Health with the powers to write those orders. At first, the board consisted of the mayor and a committee of aldermen. During epidemics of cholera and dysentery in the 1830s to 1860s, those elected officials earned a reputation as too corrupt and ineffective to protect the citizens. Quarantining ships hurt business, and as one New Yorker put it, the board was "more afraid of merchants than lying."

After the Civil War, reformers in New York State took the responsibility for health away from corrupt city politicians and gave it to an appointed Metropolitan Board of Health, requiring at least three of the nine members to be physicians. The new professional board had great power "for the purpose of preserving or protecting life or health, or preventing disease," and it could call on the city's police or its own inspectors to enforce its orders. Within a few years, the city wrested control of health back from the state, but the board kept its police powers and its professional, appointed structure. To enforce the board's orders, the city created a permanent health department, run by city's health commissioner, who also chaired the board.

After Hermann Biggs's day, the major infectious disease epidemics all but disappeared. Health departments around the country shifted to chasing less-common infectious diseases, first those preventable with vaccines, like diphtheria and whooping cough, and then those curable with antibiotics, like syphilis. To this day, every city health department has a unit to fight outbreaks of infectious diseases, no matter how small. In New York City, outbreaks of salmonella infection from contaminated food happen monthly, the mosquito-borne West Nile virus arrived in 1999, and the biggest infectious outbreak of them all, AIDS, landed in 1979. Those outbreaks can still terrify people and launch the health department into action, as when a single man was diagnosed with Ebola in New York City in 2014. One Friday in 2002, Mayor Bloomberg's chief of staff Peter Madonia glimpsed that fear. Frieden called to say, "We have somebody with bubonic plague in the hospital." Madonia said later, "I told him, 'Tom, nobody's used those words in five hundred years! What are you talking about!'"

As frightening as infectious disease outbreaks are, by the 1950s chronic diseases like heart disease and cancer were killing many more New Yorkers, so the city's health leaders had to rethink their mission. "Infectious diseases were largely under control," wrote Leona Baumgartner, the city's health commissioner from 1954 to 1962. "The limited goals of the current public health needed stretching." But because chronic diseases roused little panic, for the remainder of the century health departments received little funding to take them on. Most health departments promoted healthy behavior, usually by distributing pamphlets, but that didn't do much. In 2002 it fell to Tom Frieden to persuade people that, in this modern era, public health was still purchasable and that he knew how to buy it.

· · ·

Even before he came back to New York City, Frieden began pestering people he trusted to join him at the health department. One person dropped into his lap.

When Frieden was a medical student, he had met Colin "Coke" McCord, a chest surgeon who was the father of one of his classmates. By then McCord had spent decades on health projects in destitute areas of the world. When I first spoke to McCord in 2009, he had just returned from Tanzania, where he had been training lay health workers to do cesarean sections. At nearly eighty-one, he reminded me, with his genial manner and warm airy voice, of a left-wing Ronald Reagan. McCord had spent a short time in Vietnam in the 1960s as a civilian providing medical care to the Vietnamese, and according to a colleague, it had "radicalized" him. A few years later he abandoned his surgery practice in New York to run projects in primary medical care in India and then in Bangladesh. In 1980 he moved to Mozambique, where the socialist-inspired government, after defeating its Portuguese colonialists, was building a primary health care system.

He returned to the United States in the mid-1980s, landing at Harlem Hospital. There he quickly published a paper in the *New England Journal of Medicine* showing that African American men in Harlem had a shorter life expectancy than men in Bangladesh. Once when McCord was "kind of passing through" Nicaragua to see what the Sandinistas were up to, he bumped into Tom Frieden, who asked him to write an article for his newsletter. That led to McCord becoming a mentor to Frieden.

When Frieden took over the health department in 2002, McCord had just retired. With time on his hands, the older man called Frieden to ask if he could help. When Donna Shelley quit, Frieden asked McCord to run the antitobacco program. It was the first of several temporary positions the commissioner would assign to McCord over the next few years, calling him his "utility infielder." But others recognized that McCord acted more like a sage. Frieden could get lost in the details, but "Coke helped give Tom clarity."

"I'm good at giving advice on what to do," McCord told me, "but not so good at doing it."

Frieden also hired a young assistant, Christina Chang. The daughter of Taiwanese immigrants, Chang at first knew little about public health, but she had the brainpower and, more important, the straight-A-student eagerness for hard work and long hours that Frieden demanded. Even she found his pace tough to handle, though. Already rail thin, "I lost five pounds in the first few weeks just trying to keep up."

At the time, banning smoking in bars was a radical idea. When Chang heard Frieden's plan, "I was shocked by the ambition," she later recalled. "That's when I thought Tom was really crazy." In 1995 New York City had prohibited smoking in bigger restaurants but still allowed it in smaller restaurants, in bars, and in restaurants with their own bars. California and some towns in other states had banned smoking in bars, but in the rest of the country, bars existed almost as much for smoking as they did for drinking. But, Chang said, "I thought it wasn't my job to doubt. It was my job to try to figure out how to convince."

Frieden gathered his team and asked what arguments they needed to rebut. He intended to bring scientific data to bear on each of them. The first argument was that secondhand smoke was merely a nuisance. In fact, secondhand smoke—a mix of carbon monoxide and fine particles that are proven carcinogens—caused not just lung cancer but also heart attacks. The CDC estimated that secondhand smoke was responsible for 50,000 deaths a year nationally, which translated to more than 1,000 deaths a year in New York City. That was more than the number of city residents who died each year from homicide.

Even if the policy makers recognized that secondhand smoke was dangerous, they might reject a ban since people could just avoid smoke-filled bars. Frieden's team decided to highlight the injustice for people who didn't have that option. Waiters, waitresses, and bartenders couldn't leave when a customer lit up and couldn't afford to quit working. The team dug through scientific reports for the most powerful words to explain the risk. "Working 8 hours in a bar is equivalent to smoking 16 cigarettes," they wrote. "Bartenders have higher rates of lung cancer than firefighters and miners."

The toughest argument to rebut was that a smoke-free law would hurt the restaurant and bar business. Given the opposition that Frieden's team expected, this was also the most important one. They found numbers showing after California passed its smoke-free laws, sales in restaurants and bars—as well as the number of employees—actually grew faster.

To deflect Mayor Bloomberg's political advisers, the team produced other kinds of numbers. The nonprofit organizations that Donna Shelley had funded had commissioned a poll that showed that New York City voters liked the idea of smoke-free bars (57 percent) and loved the idea of smoke-free restaurants (84 percent). By two-to-one margins, New Yorkers said if restaurants and bars were smoke-free, they would actually be more likely to go there.

Frieden also wanted to count the number of smoking-related deaths his ban might prevent—or as he saw it, the number of lives it would save. That was the number, ultimately, that mattered most. The department's epidemiologists told him that there were just too many unknowns to make that kind of estimate. So he did what he did whenever someone gave him an answer he didn't like; he turned to someone else.

Farzad Mostashari was, like Frieden, a graduate of the CDC's Epidemic Intelligence Service program. Also like Frieden, he had spent his two EIS years as a disease detective in New York City's health department. Born in the United States, Mostashari had been raised in Iran, where as a child he witnessed the excitement of the revolution that ousted the shah. Afterward he returned to the United States and graduated magna cum laude from Harvard and Yale Medical School. He was another numbers guy, only more abstract. If posed a question, he tended to stare off into space, rub his hand over his scalp, and restate the question as something much larger. By the time he had the answer, he had invented something new.

Frieden told him, "I need a one-pager on lives saved" from the smoking ban.

"I had no fucking idea what he was talking about!" Mostashari later remembered. But after thinking about it, he was able to cobble together a mathematical model based on the impact of secondhand smoke on mortality and the difference in death rates between smokers and nonsmokers. Over the lifetimes of people who spent time in smoky places, he estimated, smoke-free air laws would prevent more than 11,000 smoking-related deaths: 4,000 in nonsmokers who would no longer breathe secondhand smoke and 7,000 in smokers who would quit. It was an odd model. Most of the lives wouldn't be saved for years. And the model counted only people who spent time in smoky workplaces in 2002, not people who would work there in the future. But it was an estimate that Frieden could defend, so he went with it.

The health commissioner then had to persuade Bloomberg's City Hall lieutenants to let him pitch the idea to the mayor. Those advisers included press officer Ed Skyler, chief of staff Peter Madonia, deputy mayor for economic development Dan Doctoroff, and deputy mayor for operations Mark Shaw. None of them questioned the health benefits. But all were dead opposed.

Ed Skyler was convinced that the public backlash would sink them. When people went to a bar, they expected others to smoke. That's what you did in a bar. Average New Yorkers would hate the law, so they would flout it, and the city wouldn't be able to enforce it.

Peter Madonia, who was managing fallout from the post-9/11 budget crisis, thought the timing couldn't have been worse. "You only have so many political chits in your honeymoon," he said years later. "Not all of us thought it was a really good idea in the context of a $7 billion dollar deficit where you're going to raise people's [property] taxes 18.5 percent, lay off sanitation workers, cut a class of cops, and close six firehouses. . . . And now you're going to tell people you can't smoke in a bar. Like, who the fuck needs this now?"

As a group, the deputy mayors believed that if the rule passed, New Yorkers who smoked would avoid the city's bars and restaurants. They'd go to Long Island or Westchester County, or they'd just stay home. Restaurants and bars in lower Manhattan closed for months after 9/11, the deputies argued, and the clubs were just now barely crawling back to life. And Frieden wanted to hit them with this? Sure, his numbers on the financial impact in California were positive, but that state was a bunch of tree-huggers.

Deputy Mayor Doctoroff even worried about tourism, especially from abroad. A tourist from Germany might pass up New York City because he couldn't smoke in a bar there. So Frieden had Chang, McCord, and others survey tour operators in each of the eight countries that sent the most visitors to New York City. The tour operators confirmed that tourists didn't ask or care about a city's smoking rules.

Doctoroff also wasn't satisfied with the data on restaurant and bar sales and employment in California. He wanted to know what happened in that state's big cities. So Frieden had his team call twenty restaurants in Los Angeles and twenty in San Francisco. More restaurants said they had seen an increase in sales after going smoke-free than a decrease.

The only person in City Hall who seemed open to the idea was Bloomberg. When Frieden finally got to him, the mayor peppered his health commissioner with questions about the data. Unlike his deputies, Bloomberg questioned the health impact, pressing on Mostashari's 11,000-lives-saved estimate. He waved off the business impact of the law in California; that state was nothing like New York City. The aides asked Frieden for other examples, but the only other examples were small towns, and comparing New York City to a small town was offensive.

At a final decision meeting, Frieden showed Bloomberg the tourism data. After all the questions to that point, at this meeting Frieden remembers the mayor asking only one: "Are you certain that this is going to save lives?" Frieden was.

Bloomberg approved it.

A long-term antismoking advocate, Joe Cherner, had anticipated this moment and had primed Frieden to steel the mayor for the battles ahead. "You can't just get him to agree," Frieden remembers Cherner saying. "You've got to tell him that he's going to be attacked. That friends are going to come up to him. That people are going to scream at him. At parties social friends, powerful people, will tell him you're doing a terrible thing. They'll tell him it's impossible." As soon as Frieden began warning Bloomberg, though, the mayor cut him off. The man who had made billions selling computer terminals told his health commissioner, "Let me tell you the first rule of salesmanship. After you make the sale, leave."

• • •

The governments of New York City and New York State are hopelessly intertwined and mutually resentful. The state is demographically lopsided: eight million of its nineteen million people live in the city, making for huge overlaps in the two governments' authority and constituencies. The city is heavily Democratic, while the rest of the state leans Republican. City officials resent the state's power over the city; the state controls much that city residents expect the mayor to manage, including the public transit system, income and sales tax rates, and pensions for city workers. City officials believe that the state sucks money from the city's business engine and showers it on economically weaker cities and towns. State officials, on the other hand, chafe when the city acts as if it were its own nation.

By state law, Mayor Bloomberg's cigarette tax increase needed approval first by the state legislature, then by the City Council. After 9/11, New York State, like neighboring Connecticut and New Jersey, had developed a deep budget hole. That helped. Legislators are always afraid of voter backlash from raising taxes, but despite the lobbying of Phillip Morris and bodega owners that sold cigarettes, they warmed up to a cigarette tax—80 percent of voters didn't smoke. All three of the region's state legislatures opened the cigarette tax spigot, but New York outdid its neighbors. The New York State legislature raised the state's own tax from $1.11 to $1.50. Then it passed the law allowing the city to increase its tax from 8 cents to $1.50, but only after grabbing 46 percent of the city's tax revenue for the state government. "Albany always screws the city, basically," said Frieden.

In June 2002 the New York City Council voted to hike the city tax, driving the total state and city tax for a pack of cigarettes in New York City from $1.19 to $3.00—by far the highest in the nation. A pack of cigarettes would soon cost over $7.00, a big hit for people buying a pack or two every day. Despite a late plea by Frieden, none of the revenue from those taxes would go to the health department to prevent smoking.

Meanwhile at the health department, Frieden was working on a different problem. The man who measured what mattered had no way of tracking year to year how many people were smoking. In April 2002 he asked Farzad Mostashari to figure out how to count smokers. Mostashari adapted a telephone survey designed by the CDC, found a call center to do it, started the calling in May, and finished surveying 10,000 people by June 30. The survey showed that 21.6 percent of adults in the city (or 1.3 million people) smoked. For the next seven years, Frieden would pay more attention to that number than any other.

• • •

Even though Frieden and his allies now had the city's executive branch behind them, they approached the passing of the Smoke-Free Air Act as if it were an insurgent political campaign. They wrote lists of influential supporters and opponents and divvied up the job of contacting them, sequencing the meetings so that they could use support from some as leverage with others. They scheduled press events and lined up people to praise the bill. They wrote scripts for ads to run on the radio, with Bloomberg and Frieden making the case, and they created print ads to run in the city's newspapers with the tagline "there's no such thing as a nonsmoking section." They paid for another poll. They made pitches to editorial boards at the city's newspapers.

They scheduled lobbying visits to all the key City Council members, assigning them according to their importance to Bloomberg or Frieden. In the heat of the election campaign, an antitobacco advocate had sent questionnaires to council candidates, asking whether they supported smoke-free restaurants and bars; now, Frieden pulled out their questionnaires, hoping to pin down those council members who had answered yes.

For the visits, Frieden's team assembled a packet with facts and numbers. A slide presentation in the packet went through twenty drafts before the commissioner was ready to show it to each of the dozen or so council members he lobbied. It was a lecture, and Frieden loved lecturing.

As they drafted the documents, the City Hall communications team choked on the phrase "Second-Hand Smoke Kills." Wasn't the word *kills* over the top? But Frieden insisted that that was just the point. They had to say it killed. If they couldn't, they would lose the argument before it started. Just before the visits, the team prepared—just in case they needed it—a pointed touch: a big bar chart showing the number of deaths they estimated were caused by smoking within each council member's district each year. The least was the district of Hiram Monserrate in Queens—85 dead. The most was the district of Domenic Recchia of Brooklyn—276 dead.

And there was one more chunk of data that Frieden wanted. He pushed his staff in the Environmental Health Division to find machines to measure how bad the air was in the city's smoky bars and, in a stroke of brilliance, to measure air quality in other nasty places for comparison. The findings couldn't have been better. Frieden was able to add a bar chart showing that "there is 50 times more air pollution in a smoky bar than in the Holland tunnel at rush hour."

On a warm day in August 2002, the team launched the Smoke-Free Air Act campaign at a press conference in City Hall Park. Bloomberg was flanked by Frieden, the head of the city's public hospital system, a few supportive restaurant and bar owners, representatives of "the A's" (American

Heart Association, American Lung Association, and the American Cancer Society), the president of the health care workers' union, the Reverend Calvin Butts, and—to add a little glamour—New York Mets pitcher Al Leiter. (Later Frieden would laugh that they had rolled out the antismoking law with "Butts and Leiter.")

"No one should have to breathe poison to hold a job," Mayor Bloomberg said. The proposed law was about much more than restaurants and bars. It would prohibit smoking in virtually every workplace, including office buildings, factories, warehouses, banks, stores, sports arenas, and transit facilities.

The City Hall team had wanted to create a splash, but they got more of a flop. The story had leaked to the papers three days before the launch, so the press ignored the unity show, but in the days beforehand the papers handed a megaphone to the opponents. Using arguments that would become familiar, they attacked the proposal as an interference with personal freedoms that would damage an industry and kill jobs. "If you can't have a cigarette in a bar," the *Times* quoted one bar patron, "what is the world coming to?" The *Post* quoted an economics professor saying that business in bars could decline 20 percent. The head of the Greater New York Restaurant and Liquor Dealers Association said, "There are going to be fights in bars and it's going to backfire and hit Bloomberg in the puss. This is a violation of people's rights. . . . What are they going to do next: come into your bedroom and tell you when to have sex?" The *Post* also went after Frieden's numbers, calling the claim that twice as many New Yorkers died from secondhand smoke as from murder "conjured up" and "nonsense on its face."

The team knew they would have to do better at the upcoming City Council hearings. The statistics might have convinced Bloomberg, but to convince the public, Christina Chang realized the team needed "the power of the anecdote." The members of the tobacco team and the antismoking advocates outside the agency were about as familiar with bars as heavy smokers are with gyms; but they began prowling bars at night, looking for bartenders, waitresses, musicians, and bouncers who had emotional stories to tell.

Frieden got crucial and early support from the chair of the City Council's health committee, Christine Quinn. The health committee had been Quinn's reward for supporting council member Gifford Miller in his run for speaker. The thirty-five-year-old daughter of a union steward steeped in city politics, Quinn was part street activist and part old-school pol. In the 1990s she had advanced from affordable-housing rabble-rouser to City Council staffer to council member and was now rising in the chamber's leadership. She was full of energy and ambition, with a big voice and a brassy laugh. Like others who succeed in politics, she could bring people around to her point of view either by charming them or by screaming at them.

Quinn cared deeply about health, for very personal reasons. Her mother, a social worker who had "always had this thing about doctors," nonetheless smoked and died of breast cancer when Christine was sixteen. "Look, if you spend one minute as a girl in the Sloan Kettering smoking lounge," she said, referring to the room where hospitalized cancer victims—in patient gowns—dragged on cigarettes, "that's all you ever need to see." When Bloomberg's political aides felt her out on the smoke-free campaign, she came back strong. "If the mayor wants to do this, I'm all in."

Before the hearings, Frieden's team strategized with Quinn about how to get the bill through. Simple and beautiful ideas, when you try to write them into law, always turn complicated and ugly. The transformation happens when you draw the lines. What should the law say about private, members-only clubs? What about outdoor patio areas? What about restaurants that had just sunk big bucks into installing ventilation systems to keep their nonsmokers happy? What about cigar bars?

Quinn scheduled two days of hearings. The first was full of entertainment. Two hours before the hearing was to begin, a huge crowd gathered in front of City Hall, as a *New York Times* reporter put it, "in a display of civic theater not seen since the AIDS protests in the early days of the Giuliani administration. Hotel workers traded barbs with bar customers, bartenders interrupted the news conferences of smoking opponents, and a man dressed as a large cigarette bobbed silently among the crowd . . . holding a placard that read, 'I ♥ secondhand smoke.'"

Inside the council chambers, Quinn had organized the speakers into panels, alternating pro and con. Leading off was a panel with Bloomberg and Frieden, Nobel Prize–winning cancer researcher Harold Varmus, and African American cocktail waitress Martinah Payne-Yehuda, whom the health team had found through their barroom carousing.

Bloomberg claimed the proposed law would "almost certainly save more lives than any other proposal that will ever come before you in this chamber. . . . The right to breathe clean air is more important than the license to pollute it." To those who suggested that the law should cover restaurants but not bars, the mayor asked, "Which workers have lives that are worth less than yours or mine?" Frieden, playing to the strong labor sentiments on the council, called the bill "a national model for worker protection—protection from deadly secondhand smoke that dispropor-tionately affects minority workers, underpaid and working long hours." Varmus testified about the medical risks of secondhand smoke.

But the most persuasive member of the panel, according to Chang, was the cocktail waitress. Payne-Yehuda had quit her job when she became pregnant because she couldn't bear the thought of exposing her baby to secondhand smoke's chemicals.

The hearing lasted over eight hours. "There were at least twenty res-taurant owners against for every one in favor," remembered Chang. The bill was unfair not just to them, the owners said, but also to their poor immigrant employees, who would lose jobs. They portrayed Bloomberg as an uncaring billionaire. "The mayor is a brilliant businessman," one owner testified, "but he knows absolutely nothing about the bar busi-ness." "It was ugly," said Frieden. "It was very ugly."

Before and after the hearings, the bars lobbied hard, both in the press and behind the scenes. "They had spent a lot of money supporting candi-dates," said Bloomberg chief of staff Madonia. "So this was their moment to call in their chits. And they did, believe me."

"It was a huge fight on a host of different levels," said Christine Quinn. "The restaurants and the bars, in a way that is hard to imagine now, turned out in total force." The council members listened to them and grew nervous. "It was venturing into the unknown."

Quinn held firm, though. Despite the pressure, Frieden's team thought they had the votes they needed. But the bill wouldn't come up for a vote without the blessing of Gifford Miller, the council speaker. Bloomberg had talked to him early on and told reporters that he had his support, but Miller publicly backed off from the bill and privately was cagey. "Quinn was terrific, steadfast," recalled Frieden. But he didn't trust Miller.

Negotiators in the City Council and the mayor's office haggled over possible compromises to address thorny situations and to placate those who were waffling. "We had tons and tons of meetings with the restaurants, who wanted all kinds of exemptions," Quinn said later. The mayor's staff agreed to grandfather a handful of specialty cigar bars. They would allow smoking in the few private "owner-operated bars." They would permit smoking in outdoor sidewalk cafés, but only in separate smoking sections with at least three feet of buffer.

But when it came to the major change that the opponents wanted—allowing separate smoking rooms in bars—Frieden dug in his heels. The tobacco companies were pushing fancy ventilation systems, saying they would protect nonsmokers in nearby rooms. Even high-powered ventilation systems, though, only got rid of the secondhand smoke smell; they didn't clean out enough of the fine particles to protect lungs. And workers in bars with smoking rooms would have to enter these rooms to serve customers.

The biggest danger of separate smoking rooms, and the reason the tobacco companies liked them, was something the health team didn't want to talk much about: if bars could have separate smoking rooms, then other businesses—like restaurants, movie theaters, and offices—would demand them, too. A comprehensive smoke-free law would help make smoking socially unacceptable, but allowing public places to have separate smoking rooms could create new "cool" places to hang out in, which could do just the opposite.

According to Frieden, Speaker Miller was demanding the separate rooms, or he would not allow the bill to come up for a vote. After all their work, the bill looked like it was dying: "Negotiations collapsed . . .

we were going to give up because [Miller] wouldn't move it." Miller may have privately sided with bar owners. But he would need help from the mayor on many issues for the rest of his four-year term as speaker. And Bloomberg was determined; he had told Peter Madonia that the smoking ban was one of only two legislative acts he really wanted, the other being mayoral control of the school system.

In early December 2002, four months after the mayor announced the bill and two months after the hearings, Bloomberg and Miller walked into a meeting room in City Hall. They spoke for about fifteen minutes alone. Frieden and his team hovered anxiously outside. Afterward the two men walked out and passed the health team, saying nothing. Within a few days, though, Frieden got his orders: create an option in the law for bars to build separate smoking rooms, but according to your specifications.

On the surface, it looked like Frieden had lost. But "specifications" gave him leverage. He was a tuberculosis expert, after all, who had taught hospital administrators how to build "respiratory isolation" rooms for TB patients. So his specs for smoking rooms were powerful enough to protect anyone from tuberculosis. The rooms must have "negative air pressure," so air would only flow in from other areas and then be sucked directly outdoors, vented twenty-five feet from any air intake grate. The rooms couldn't take up more than one-fourth of the club's floor space. They had to have their own sprinkler systems. The owners could not offer food or drinks inside, and they had to post signs saying that employees couldn't enter the rooms. "You're basically building a plastic phone booth in the middle of your restaurant or bar," said Chang. To top it off, Frieden added a sunset: after three years, the smoking rooms would shut down.

The phone-booth smoking rooms fooled no one. At another raucous day of hearings, one council member said, "the thing that I think is the most appalling to me is the fraudulence of this compromise. . . . I haven't met anybody who has read through these regulations and realistically thinks anybody's going to be able to build a room in their bar."

The vote the next week was 42 to 7 in favor. New York City would have smoke-free workplaces, including all bars and restaurants, beginning in March 30, 2003.

Years later Christine Quinn said that Gifford Miller had intended to allow the bill to pass all along. "I know Gifford was not going to let it die," she said. "It was not a burning issue for him, but it was a burning issue for me . . . and he was not going to leave me hanging." But "he was going to get what he could get for it." According to Quinn, what Miller got from Bloomberg was a promise not to veto a bill that Miller favored raising the minimum wage for home health care workers.

Michael Bloomberg signed the Smoke-Free Air Act into law on December 30, 2002, nearly a year to the day after he took office. At the ceremony in City Hall, he again cited Frieden's numbers: "This bill will free more than 400,000 non-smoking New Yorkers from exposure to cancer-causing chemicals and will save more than 11,000 lives in New York City over the life of the law. New York City is the greatest city in the world. . . . And with the passage of this statute, we go a long way toward becoming one of the healthiest cities as well."

3

"I thought, this nutrition stuff is so controversial."

Mary Bassett is a slender woman with a habit of parking her glasses in the graying curls on top of her head when she looks up from reading. She speaks as calmly and carefully as a diplomat, but her words are strong and often about injustice. When I first met her, she had framed on her office wall a ballot from South Africa's 1994 election with Nelson Mandela's name on it and a quote from Dante: "The hottest places in hell are reserved for those who, in a time of great moral crisis, maintain their neutrality."

Bassett's father had overcome historic barriers to give Mary the life he couldn't have himself. Emmett Bassett, an African American, came from a family of subsistence farmers in Virginia. He excelled enough in school to make it to the Tuskegee Institute, studying under George Washington Carver. When he was drafted into the army in World War II, he was assigned to a blacks-only unit. After talking to the northerners he met there, he realized how limited even his college education was, so afterward he went back to school, earning a Ph.D. in biochemistry. He took a job as a professor at a medical school in Newark, settled into the Washington Heights section of Manhattan with his wife, a librarian who was white, and sent his children to a private school with children of investment bankers. It was a great school, and his daughter Mary wasn't bothered by being one of the few nonwhite children there, but she did resent thinking that, next to her classmates, she was poor. "We were not poor," she told me emphatically. "I *felt* we were, but we were not poor." Her parents were deeply rooted civil rights activists. "As far back as I can remember, we children were carted along to marches and meetings," she wrote in a short autobiography in a book called *Comrades in Health*.

At Radcliffe, Mary Bassett volunteered at the Black Panther Free Clinic in Boston, going door to door in the surrounding ghetto to test children for sickle cell disease. After graduating with honors, she came back to New York City for medical school and chose to do her residency at Harlem Hospital. When she finished her training, she was drawn to the African liberation movement, so she headed to Zimbabwe during "the exhilarating post-independence 1980s." She joined the medical faculty at the University of Zimbabwe in Harare just when AIDS began ravaging that country.

In the university's hospital, she told "hundreds and hundreds of people that they were HIV-infected." "There were lots of fairly wrenching human stories," she remembered years later, including a young guy who was a personal secretary to the president. "I guess by now he's dead." She traveled to factories and schools to educate people about AIDS and the risks of having unprotected sex. Thinking back on it, she felt most of her efforts had failed. Because she had no treatment to offer those who were infected, "denial was the most effective response." That was okay for their psyche, but it did nothing to stop the spread of the virus to others. "Zimbabwe went on to have one of the worst epidemics of the continent," she told me, because they weren't fixing the root social problems. "In retrospect, I think we were trying to solve a cholera epidemic by teaching schoolchildren how to wash their hands."

Bassett had heard of Coke McCord at Harlem Hospital but hadn't met him. She had a chance one time when she traveled from Zimbabwe to Mozambique. Arriving in Maputo, she went to the hospital and asked in broken Spanish if Dr. McCord was on the grounds. The hospital workers ushered her into an operating suite, where McCord was in full surgeon's scrubs, plunging his hands into a patient's open chest to strip off a diseased heart lining. Most surgeons would have been apoplectic to be interrupted by a woman in street clothes while holding a scalpel inches from a beating heart, but McCord acted as calmly as if he were changing a tire. After asking who she was, he told her he was nearly finished and, if she'd wait outside, he'd be happy to chat later.

Many Americans who feel called to do medical work in the world's poor countries stick it out for a year or two. Mary Bassett's time in Zimbabwe, interrupted by stints in the United States, stretched to seventeen. But as the AIDS epidemic raged in that country through the 1990s, the political and economic conditions also went into a death spiral. The World Bank and the IMF demanded a "structural adjustment" for Zimbabwe, which forced the government to deregulate prices and spend less on health care.

This requirement not only devastated the clinics but also triggered a much larger unraveling. Robert Mugabe, the nation's founding father, grabbed total power. He repressed his political opponents, provoked violent takeovers of white-owned farms, engaged in a war in neighboring Congo, and began printing massive amounts of currency, spawning a withering hyperinflation. Bassett's hospital fell apart, with doctors disappearing to work elsewhere and patients' families having to pay in cash in advance for everything from medicine to IV tubing. One day a story appeared in the paper that the government was investigating a human rights group for which Bassett was a board member. That was enough. A friend who knew Tom Frieden from "the TB wars" told her that he was going to lead the New York City health department, so she wrote him a letter.

When Bassett first met Frieden in late 2002, during the peak of the smoke-free-air fight, she found him "very cocky." She knew her résumé was unusual. But she thought Frieden might value her many years working outside the U.S. system, because "it was clear that he had come in with an intent to shake things up." She was right. He offered her the chance to run the agency's AIDS program.

Surprisingly, Bassett turned him down. She wanted to work on the diseases that mattered most, and in New York, AIDS wasn't the biggest killer. She thought back on her time at Harlem Hospital, where "I don't think I've ever seen sicker people." They were suffering and dying not from infections but from chronic diseases, like heart disease and cancer and kidney failure. "In Zimbabwe I saw very sick people, but usually they had one condition that was life-threatening. But in Harlem the problem list was always eight problems long."

So despite her limited experience, she asked Frieden if instead she could direct the department's work to prevent chronic diseases. She was surprised when he agreed, offering her the new job of deputy commissioner for the Division of Health Promotion and Disease Prevention, which he had formed by merging a community health unit with a few other programs, including tobacco. She worried about how well she would tolerate Frieden's style, but she jumped in anyway.

The biggest health problem the division faced was heart disease. Even if the health department were to erase smoking from New York City, 17,000 New Yorkers would still die from heart disease each year—more than were killed by all types of cancer combined. Tom Frieden, steeped from childhood in medical care, wanted to prevent heart disease by getting doctors to treat three major risk factors: diabetes, high blood pressure, and high blood cholesterol.

It infuriated him that the American medical care system could perform heart transplants but couldn't do the simple things that would prevent people from needing them. A slide that he showed in many lectures read, "On ABC's of health care, USA gets an 'F.'" Doctors treated effectively only one-third of Americans with high blood pressure (the B in ABC), one-fourth of Americans with diabetes (the A, for the hemoglobin A1C test), and one-tenth of Americans with high blood cholesterol (the C). To Frieden, that meant the health department should coax or shame doctors into providing better preventive care, and that it should push people to go to doctors and take their pills.

Medical treatment of risk factors is known as "secondary prevention." At the time, though, many in public health were shifting toward "primary prevention," or helping people avoid diabetes, high blood pressure, and high cholesterol in the first place. The basic idea of primary prevention is simple: people need to eat healthier food—more fruits and vegetables and less salt, sugar, and fat—and exercise more. But making that happen across a whole city of eight million was more than daunting. When doctors try to persuade even one person to behave differently, they usually fail. Public health agencies did what they could with health education and promotion for the whole population, but they barely scratched the surface of the problem.

Mary Bassett had ideas for a third way. She appeared at her first staff meeting waving graphs drawn by the British preventive medicine specialist Geoffrey Rose. The Rose graphs, shaped like bell curves, illustrated a population's behavior, such as the number of calories people took in. Health educators found people on the risky tail of the curve (the people who ate much more than average) and cajoled them to join the less-risky people in the center (by eating less). It didn't work very well. The educators reached only a few people, and only a fraction of those could overcome the pressures of life to alter their daily habits. But Rose thought prevention experts should instead shift the entire curve—getting everyone to eat just a little bit less—by changing the everyday world around people. "This is what we're going to do," Bassett announced. "We're going to shift curves."

She saw traditional health promotion as blaming the victim—lecturing poor people who were adapted to horrible circumstances that they, rather than their circumstances, were the problem. She was determined that "we weren't going to have a whole health promotion and disease prevention division that was aimed at imploring people to do better." She wanted to fix the social injustices that made people eat wrong. Among other radical changes, that meant she needed very different types of people working in the division. "I'm proud to say that not a single person that I recruited to the division had a formal background in health promotion."

When she got into the job, Bassett discovered that the health department was already shifting curves in the way it fought smoking. The cigarette taxes and the Smoke-Free Air Act didn't entreat people to resist an unhealthy world or scold them if they couldn't resist. Instead, those policies made healthy choices easier and unhealthy choices harder. She wanted to do the same for eating.

But eating is much more complicated than smoking. To a doctor, smoking is an absolute evil. No one should smoke, ever. That means that tighter regulations on cigarettes, from smoke-free-air laws to high taxes, are always better. But no food is as toxic as tobacco, and everyone has to eat. And there are so many different kinds of problems with Americans' diet. People don't eat enough fruits or vegetables. They eat too much saturated fat, too much salt, and too much sugar, and—as is painfully obvious from the obesity epidemic—they consume too many calories.

America's food system, which shapes the American diet, is gigantic and complicated. Food flows from farms and factories into people's mouths not only through grocery stores but also through corner stores (which New Yorkers call bodegas), restaurants, fast-food joints, school cafeterias, bookstores, snack counters, vending machines, and food banks. Every year the channels grew and diversified. How could one health department alter that deluge of mostly unhealthy food? Even if it was willing to start with one tiny stream, which one would it be?

Coke McCord, who now reported to Mary Bassett, surprised her with a suggestion. He had read *Eat, Drink, and Be Healthy* by Walter Willett, head of nutrition at the Harvard School of Public Health. "Read this," he said, passing the book on to her. "Then we can talk about trans fat."

Trans fats are chemicals that are literally twists on natural oils. No matter what people say, they love the taste of fat. They put butter on bread, pour cream into their coffee, lap up ice cream, and layer nearly everything with cheese. But butterfat is expensive to produce, turns rancid if left at room temperature, and burns too easily when cooked. In 1901 a German chemist showed that if he combined vegetable oil with hydrogen gas and metallic nickel at temperatures approaching one thousand degrees, he could transform it into a semisolid fat. The artificial fat didn't turn bad if left in a kitchen cabinet, and it didn't burn as easily.

A few years later Procter and Gamble bought the patent rights to his "partial hydrogenation" process and used it to turn cottonseed oil into a white solid fat that the company sold as "shortening" under the name

Crisco. Not long afterward food companies added flavoring and yellow coloring to "partially hydrogenated vegetable oil" and sold it as a butter substitute that they called oleomargarine. By the 1960s, artificial trans fats lurked nearly everywhere in American grocery stores, appearing not just in margarine and frying oils but also in cookies, crackers, pastries, pizza crusts, candy bars, mayonnaise, and peanut butter. For decades, few questioned what trans fats did inside the humans who ate them. The fats predated the Food and Drug Administration (FDA), and when it was founded, the FDA grandfathered trans fats in as "generally recognized as safe."

But in the 1980s researchers began discovering that trans fats are in fact toxic. First, studies showed that eating them raised blood cholesterol levels even more than consuming the same amount of cholesterol or saturated fat. Then Walter Willett's research group at Harvard, as well as others, repeatedly found that people who eat more trans fats are more likely to have heart attacks. Eating just 4 grams a day—the amount in a typical order of French fries—increases the risk of coronary heart disease by 23 percent. And Americans on average were eating more trans fats than that every day. Chris Gallin, whose heart attack nearly killed him at age forty-six, loved French fries and ate two slices of pizza every day for lunch. By 1994 Willett's group estimated that at least 30,000 Americans died every year from heart disease caused by trans fats.

Stalin is reputed to have said that the death of one man is a tragedy but the death of millions is a statistic. No one sees the sad reality of this psychology more than those who work in public health. Teams of doctors and nurses may work around the clock in an ICU to save the life of a single person from a heart attack; anyone who suggests they are wasting their effort is seen as cruel. But for many years, few people paid any attention to the 30,000-deaths-per-year toll from trans fats.

In the early 2000s, under pressure from nutrition activists, the FDA was finally considering a minimal rule that would require food companies to list trans fats on packages' Nutrition Facts panels. But how many people would flip over a box of crackers to see if they contained trans fats? Also, food at restaurants wasn't labeled.

With all the city's nutritional problems, trans fats might seem a strange place for the health department to start. But public health, like politics, is the art of the possible. To McCord, trans fats were a great target because like tobacco (and unlike salt, sugar, or natural saturated fats) they were pure evil—artificial, unnecessary, and killing people by the tens of thousands. McCord argued that the city should just ban trans fats—they should never have been allowed in food the first place. The team was inspired in mid-2003 when Denmark passed a trans fats ban, the first country to do so.

Bassett and McCord took the idea to the department's chief lawyer, Wilfredo Lopez. Could the Board of Health ban trans fats? they asked.

The Board of Health hadn't changed its structure much since the late 1800s, despite many revisions of the New York City Charter. It now had eleven appointed members with expertise in health, five of whom by charter rules were physicians.

Lopez told Mary Bassett no. The Board of Health regulated what happened in restaurant kitchens to avoid bacterial contamination of food. "Historically, we didn't get into the business of the content of the food," he told me later. That was the FDA's job. "As long as it wasn't poisonous or declared to be a hazardous substance," he couldn't see the board banning it.

• • •

Meanwhile Frieden was learning that getting doctors to treat their patients for the disease "smoking" was hard. His newsletter warning doctors about malpractice didn't seem to change what they did. The city's Health and Hospitals Corporation should have provided him an opportunity. HHC was a behemoth, a sprawling network of eleven public hospitals and dozens of clinics. Frieden didn't run it, but he was on the board, so in theory he had influence there.

The HHC hospitals ran smoking cessation clinics, but the results were pitiful. Frieden estimated that every quarter 115,000 smokers visited doctors within the mammoth system, but only about 2,000—less than 2 percent—ended up in the cessation clinics. A report that he requested offered a long list of reasons: doctors didn't refer patients to the clinics, patients had trouble getting there, the patients spoke Spanish but the counselors didn't, there was no budget for brochures, and patients' insurance didn't pay for the medications.

Both Frieden and HHC's president wanted the health care system to do better. Urged on both by Frieden and by their own supervisors, more doctors began referring smoking patients to the cessation clinics, and the clinics did a better job of treating them—teaching them ways to quit and giving them nicotine patches and other medications that roughly doubled the quit rate. By late 2004, the clinics had tripled the number of smokers they were seeing, and about 90 percent of those seen received medications. Still, that amounted to only about 5,500 smokers every quarter—less than half a percent of smokers citywide. "That was a searing experience," Frieden said years later. "No matter how hard you pushed on cessation, you never moved the number."

So in the spring of 2003, Frieden decided to leapfrog the doctors and give medications straight to smokers. He got a donation of tens of thousands of nicotine patches and sent out a press release announcing six weeks of free patches (which otherwise cost over $100 each) for smokers who called the city's new 311 information line. Answering the calls and shipping the patches nearly overwhelmed his small tobacco team, but by the time the giveaway ended, they had mailed patches to 34,000 smokers. Six months later Frieden had his team survey 1,300 smokers who had received the patches and 160 smokers who had asked for patches but never got them. Amazingly, one-third of those who had got the patches had quit, compared to only 6 percent of those who never got them. The team estimated that the giveaways had caused 6,000 smokers to quit. That was more quitters than all of HHC's smoking cessation clinics produced in a year, at a fraction of the cost. But even that success was bittersweet, because Frieden wanted to reach all 1.3 million of the city's smokers. If he ran the patch giveaway twice a year, reaching them all would take more than a hundred years.

The Smoke-Free Air Act, on the other hand, was working far better than anyone had hoped. The panic about it had continued up until the day it went into effect. Smokers like Chris Gallin, who at that point had not yet had his heart attack, were outraged: "We felt our life was going to end." Others had predicted that bars and restaurants would just ignore the rule, or if not, that bars would roil with fights between bouncers and smokers. They were wrong. Most bars and restaurants put up no-smoking signs and began enforcing the ban on the day it went into effect. While some customers grumbled, nearly all smokers just held off while they were eating dinner or drinking and then took their puffs outdoors. Some admitted that the rule cut down their smoking and might help them quit. Later Chris Gallin said, "I hated the smoking ban, and I think it was one of the greatest things [the Bloomberg administration] ever did."

By the fourth month after the law went into effect, of fifteen hundred bars and restaurants inspected by the health department, only twenty were found breaking the rules. As people became accustomed to the clean air in restaurants and bars, polls showed support for the law rising to 62 percent. Meanwhile, despite the predictions of doom, sales in restaurants and bars actually rose 9 percent. And the city's higher cigarette tax (even after the state took half the revenue) was bringing in $130 million per year to the city.

But the most stunning numbers came from Mostashari's telephone surveys. The percent of adults in New York City who smoked fell from 21.6 percent in 2002 (before the big tax increase and the Smoke-Free Air Act) to 19.2 percent in 2003. That amounted to a drop of nearly 140,000 smokers in a single year. At first Frieden wasn't sure whether to believe it. Could the tax increase and the smoking ban have been so traumatic that a small city's worth of smokers quit almost at once? On the 2003 survey, the health department had asked former smokers why they had quit. Based on their answers, Frieden's team estimated that 59,000 former smokers credited the tax increase for their quitting, 13,000 the Smoke-Free Air Act, and 16,000 both. Maybe the plummeting smoking rate wasn't a fluke.

Many people in public health would have celebrated privately and waited another year to see if the smoking drop continued. Frieden instead declared victory immediately. His team published three papers, one describing the campaign to pass the Smoke-Free Air Act, one showing how well the nicotine patch giveaway worked, and one summarizing the success of the overall smoking program. In the third article, he wrote that "because roughly one-third of smokers die prematurely from tobacco-related disease, this decline, if sustained, will result in 45,000 fewer premature deaths."

· · ·

Lynn Silver doesn't look the slightest bit like a militant. A sandy-haired woman in her fifties who speaks softly and giggles frequently, she could be a Cub Scout den mother. One of her staff nicknamed her "Mama Bear." But underneath that manner she is tenacious, and she proved to be an unrelenting warrior on unhealthy food.

Silver was from New York but began traveling to Latin America to agitate for health even before finishing medical school at Johns Hopkins. She landed in Nicaragua two days after the Sandinista revolution in 1979 and immediately found herself "running a network of community health workers." While in Central America she ran into "a youngster at Columbia" named Tom Frieden, who was putting out his health newsletter. After a stint with the Pan American Health Organization, she signed on with Public Citizen, the advocacy organization founded by Ralph Nader. Silver was in the Health Research Group, which was directed Sidney Wolfe, a scathing critic of drug companies and the FDA. In her job interview, Wolfe asked her, "Are you prepared to work nights and weekends and Sundays and be excoriated in the press?" Silver was. During her time there she wrote muckraking pieces on the high rates of cesarean sections and took the federal government to task for allowing drug companies to charge it exorbitant rates for AIDS drugs that the government itself had paid to develop.

After spending some years in Brazil, where she taught food and drug law at a university, Silver wanted to come back to New York. She sent her résumé to Mary Bassett, who hired her in early 2004 to become her assistant commissioner for chronic diseases.

While the city bureaucracy churned through the hiring paperwork,

Bassett paid Silver as a consultant to develop a strategic plan to prevent chronic diseases. Silver's plan showed that she also had very different ideas from Tom Frieden. Like Bassett, she thought it was wrong to blame people for making unhealthy choices. People were just behaving normally in an unhealthy world. The source of Americans' unhealthy eating habits was a toxic "food environment"—a world bursting with alluring, processed, junky food. The health department needed to push for the "gradual elimination of . . . a 'toxic environment.'"

Unlike the health department's other doctors, Silver had legal skills, self-taught from her time at Public Citizen, that could transform vague concepts into concrete proposals. In her plan, she offered a long list of provocative ideas to create a healthier environment in New York City, including changing zoning requirements to encourage more supermarkets in poor neighborhoods, forcing grocery stores to stock healthier items, taxing soda and snack foods, "evaluat[ing] food/calorie labeling on restaurant menus," and "work[ing] toward smaller portion sizes in industrialized foods and in restaurants."

As radical as the plan was, it said nothing about trans fats. When Bassett asked her about them, Silver later said, "my first challenge was figuring out what trans fats were."

Around the time Lynn Silver arrived, General Counsel Wilfredo Lopez had begun a task that only Frieden would have assigned him: to update the city's health code, the compilation of Board of Health regulations. The code was the size of the Bible and about as well organized. The board had added layers upon layers of rules since the 1800s. It banned spitting (1800s), required that cases of syphilis be reported (1920s), regulated swimming pools (1960s), and specified testing procedures for HIV (1980s). It hadn't been overhauled in fifty years.

Lopez asked all the department's assistant commissioners for ideas on what should be revised. With Silver he got more than he bargained for. Lopez, she later recalled, "wanted to know whether we should get rid of the chapter that says if you go to Weight Watchers, you had to have a doctor's note." But when she learned about the health code, "a light bulb went on in my head." It was just the tool the department needed to clean up the toxic environment. The code was purely about health, it was enforced by the health department, and—most important—it was written by the Board of Health, which was insulated from political pressures. The city charter even said that the board could write health code rules to control "chronic diseases and conditions hazardous to life and health"—that is, for more than just infectious diseases. The board had used that authority in 1960 to ban lead paint in homes and in 1976 to require landlords to install window guards in buildings to protect toddlers from falls, and the state courts had upheld its authority.

Unlike Lopez, Lynn Silver was convinced that the board had the power to ban trans fats in restaurants, even if trans fats weren't declared a hazardous substance. The FDA regulated packaged food but left restaurants to states and cities. Silver believed the board could add a ban on trans fats to the restaurant section of the health code.

Silver knew how to argue with lawyers, but took another tack. She figured that if Tom Frieden wanted to rid the city's restaurants of trans fats, Wilfredo Lopez would take another look at the health code. So while talking with Lopez, she also pushed Frieden.

It took some work. At first Frieden was unimpressed with trans fats. "I thought it was hype," he said. On top of that, it didn't mesh with his doctorly instincts to just give people medicines to bring down their cholesterol. "I thought, this nutrition stuff is so controversial," he groaned.

The way to convince Frieden was with data. The job of marshaling the data fell mainly to Sonia Angell, whom Mary Bassett and Lynn Silver hired to be their director of cardiovascular disease prevention. Angell was nearly a generation younger than Bassett and two generations younger than Coke McCord. In college, Angell had majored in journalism and political science, with the career dream of making documentaries on human rights violations. After spending two years as a Peace Corps volunteer and two more as a community organizer, she decided health was her calling. She went back to school, got degrees in medicine and public health, and after her residency studied for two years with academic "social epidemiologists." She was too much of an activist to become a researcher, though.

Angell quickly became the department's expert on trans fats. She studied not just health effects but also food technology, telling Christina Chang at one point, "I can't believe I went to medical school and I know this much about pies." She and Silver fed Frieden a fat binder full of scientific papers on trans fats. He devoured the studies, puzzling over the fine print of their methods, contemplating the details, and probing the researchers' conclusions. Angell and Silver "kept briefing me and briefing me and briefing me," he said. Finally, he was convinced: trans fats kill.

But two questions loomed. First, if the health department banned trans fats, would restaurants switch to saturated fats, which might be worse? Second, could restaurants make the food that New Yorkers were accustomed to with trans-fat-free oils and spreads? The data Angell showed Frieden convinced him that the first question was moot. In feeding studies, eating trans fats raised "bad" cholesterol and lowered "good" cholesterol, while eating saturated fats raised both. "You can replace trans fats with lard and do better," Frieden said. On the second question, Frieden read the papers but was finally persuaded by a story. Bloomberg's chief of staff Peter Madonia came from a family that ran a Bronx bakery known for its cannoli. Frieden asked him how hard it would be for the bakery to get rid of trans fats. A couple of weeks later Madonia reported back that "it was not complicated at all."

Sonia Angell had to figure out if the city's restaurant suppliers had enough trans-fat-free products to meet demand. So she, Gail Goldstein (whom she had hired), and a few interns called every restaurant supply company they could reach in the city—more than a hundred of them—and asked about oils, shortening, and spreads. What they heard was surprising. Plenty of trans-fat-free "fry oils" were available, but many suppliers didn't stock them because restaurants weren't asking for them. Trans-fat-free shortening for baking might be a little harder to find, but new oils and fats were coming on the market, and the supply could quickly catch up with any increased demand.

Angell also needed to know how many of the city's thousands of restaurants cooked with trans fats. So Gail Goldstein had the health department's 150 restaurant inspectors, while checking for mice and faulty refrigerators, poke into pantries to study labels for cooking oils, hamburger buns, pie crusts, and pancake mixes. Inspectors found the words *partially hydrogenated* on labels in about half the restaurants.

Lynn Silver thought the survey showed that the restaurants could handle a ban. After all, half the restaurants already weren't using trans fats, and they were doing just fine. With Frieden now interested, Wilfredo Lopez took another look. "It took me a long time to get Wilfredo on board with these alternative uses of the code," said Silver. He still worried that the city might lose a lawsuit over a ban, but he finally came around.

Still, Frieden felt he couldn't drop a ban on trans fats on the city without first asking restaurants to give them up voluntarily. By then it was 2005, and Bloomberg would soon run for reelection; no one wanted the mayor's campaign hobbled by attacks over trans fats. Silver, convinced that a ban was necessary, nonetheless saw advantages of starting with something voluntary. If none of the restaurants dropped trans fats, it would prove that the ban was necessary. If many restaurants dropped them, it would prove that trans fats weren't needed and would justify the ban so that the rest would follow.

Angell and her team wrote letters and brochures for suppliers, restaurants, and city residents with the same message: trans fats cause heart disease, the city's biggest killer, so get rid of them. In August 2005, after nearly three years of thinking and planning, they mailed the brochures to 20,000 restaurants, 14,000 suppliers and supermarkets, and some 100,000 citizens. Angell said, "We were sending letters to Iowa—or wherever they were—saying 'by the way, in New York City we are asking that restaurants eliminate the use of artificial trans fats.'" At the same time they released a training program on trans fats for restaurant staff that ultimately was completed by 7,000 workers. They sent out a press release announcing both the mailing and the training program. The release included a quote from E. Charles Hunt, the executive vice president of the New York State Restaurant Association, about how they were "working together to reduce trans fat from our kitchens." This was the last time Hunt would say the restaurant association and Bloomberg's health department were "working together" on anything.

4

"We were failing and
we didn't know why, and
we had to succeed."

When Tom Frieden saw the smoking rate for 2005, he was stunned. It was 18.9 percent, up from 18.5 percent the year before. The uptick could have been statistical noise, but he couldn't accept that. The year before, seeing the 18.5 percent number (down 0.8 percent and 50,000 smokers from the year before that) had been "the high point of the year" for him. At a dinner at Gracie Mansion that night, he excitedly wrote the number on a napkin and passed it to Bloomberg. He was certain then that the smoking rate would keep falling. But now Frieden had to face the awful possibility that the win had been only temporary: "We were failing and we didn't know why, and we had to succeed."

He remembered from his "round table" three years earlier that the Massachusetts health department people had touted their antismoking TV ads. For nearly a century, the tobacco companies had sold cigarettes with advertising that showed smokers as sexy, sophisticated, and independent—think the Marlboro man and the Virginia Slims woman. "Counter-advertisements" were meant to replace those images in people's minds with the far uglier truth about smoking.

Almost no health departments were running counter-ads on television in 2005, but it was an old idea. In 1967 the Federal Communications Commission decided to apply its Fairness Doctrine—designed to present alternative opinions on contentious issues—to cigarette ads. It had forced television and radio stations to air one counter-ad for free for every three cigarette ads. Unlike standard public service announcements, these counter-ads ran in prime time. Over the next three years, per capita cigarette sales in the United States had fallen 7 percent. With that, the tobacco companies suddenly had a change of heart. They volunteered for a congressional ban on cigarette ads on television and radio; that action wiped out the counter-ads too, after which cigarette sales bounced back up. The lesson some antismoking advocates took was that public health agencies could win with counter-ads even if the tobacco companies outspent them. As one advocate put it, "It's easier to sell the truth than to sell a lie."

In the 1970s and 1980s researchers in California, Australia, and South Africa ran three very similar studies to test more scientifically whether counter-ads worked. Each study was done in a group of three small towns. Residents of one town saw antismoking counter-ads, those in a second town saw those ads and also received in-person antismoking education, and those in a third "control" town got neither. All three studies found that smoking rates fell faster in the counter-ad towns than in the control towns. (In two of the studies, the community programs helped cut smoking rates further.) Health departments in the United States didn't act on these studies, but public health agencies in Sydney and Melbourne, Australia, followed up with citywide campaigns, and in both cities smoking rates fell within six months. In the late 1990s, the Australian government expanded them into a national TV campaign. At about the same time, state health departments in Massachusetts and Florida began running TV ads aimed at teenagers, and in both states smoking rates fell among teens who saw the ads.

Frieden came to his role skeptical that education could change behavior, and he wasn't completely persuaded by the smoking campaign evaluations. Still, he felt he had to give counter-ads a try. That meant paying for ad time; there was no point to public service announcements airing at three a.m. "I'm going to run ten million dollars of counter-advertising and see what happens," he later recalled thinking. "It was done very specifically as an empirical experiment." By holding down hiring, he was able to bank the money he needed, but because of government budgeting rules, he had to spend it within six months. He sent his staff on a search for ads. The CDC kept a trove of antismoking TV ads and shipped them a big box of VHS tapes and DVDs.

The people who watched those first ads came from worlds very different from those of Frieden's doctors. Jeffrey Escoffier, who had directed the department's health media and marketing unit for many years, had the most unusual background. Trained as an economist, Escoffier had authored five books, ranging from a biography of John Maynard Keynes to a history of gay pornography (entitled *Bigger Than Life*). He was in his sixties and usually wore black shirts and gray ties, which with his gray beard gave him the look of an aging revolutionary, but he was actually mild-mannered, sunny, and curious. Sarah Perl, who ran the Bureau of Tobacco Control, had the tough, hurried manner of a newspaper reporter, which she had been for years.

Escoffier and Perl had to choose which ads in the CDC's box—if any—were worth spending millions of dollars on airing. All smokers know that smoking is bad for their health, but they find creative reasons to deny that it matters. The ads tried different ways to make the risk immediate and personal. The Australian campaign attacked the excuse that it takes decades for smoking to kill you. *Every Cigarette Is Doing You Damage* showed young people inhaling deep drags of smoke and then followed that smoke into their bodies and the organs that it damaged. Hands wearing latex surgeons' gloves opened body organs on screen—a brain oozing blood from a stroke, a lung with a year's worth of tar poured over it, an aorta out of which the hands squeezed a snake of yellow cholesterol goo.

The Massachusetts ads, by contrast, were testimonials. A man named Mike Sams told how it felt to be dying of lung cancer at thirty-seven. A woman named Pam Laffin, her face moonlike and pink from steroid treatments, was suffering after a lung transplant in her twenties. "Oh my god, the fear of breathing, or not being able to breathe, is worse than anything in the world," she tells the viewer. At the end the text appears silently, "Pam died of emphysema." Another featured a man who was not dying. Ronaldo Martinez, stricken with throat cancer at age thirty, had a tracheotomy—a hole in his throat—and without a larynx spoke in a computerized monotone using an electronic gadget he held to his neck. The ad showed him protecting his tracheotomy while taking a shower so the water didn't choke him, then cleaning and dressing it afterward. "Nothing will ever be the same again," his computer voice says. "Not even the simple things."

Studying the ads forced Escoffier and Perl to consider whether they wanted negative or positive messages. The Australian and Massachusetts ads tried to scare smokers into quitting. But as Escoffier explained to me later, advertising had always been seen as "aspirational." Commercial ads sell Pepsi, pickup trucks, and lipstick by linking them to ideas and feelings that we cherish, like happiness, friendship, respect, and love. Health educators, in a very different world from commercial advertisers, accept as gospel that "scare tactics don't work." Escoffier's earlier campaigns had all been positive, selling the good life that comes from healthy actions.

With no time to spare, Perl and Escoffier ran the negative ads anyway. They aired *Every Cigarette Is Doing You Damage* just after Christmas 2005 and followed up with Pam Laffin and Mike Sams. As they were running them, they hired an advertising agency to come up with other ideas. The agency's first try took a positive tack. *Everybody Loves a Quitter* showed how much smokers' children, parents, and spouses would appreciate them if they gave up smoking. "My man," a woman says, giving her husband a hug. "A quitter—that's so sexy. Mmmm."

Perl and Escoffier asked Beth Kilgore to test the ads with smokers, testing that was too late for this round but might teach them something for future campaigns. Kilgore is a quiet and thoughtful woman, trained as a sociologist to do qualitative research, who worked in Farzad Mostashari's epidemiology unit. When she started, she admitted, "We didn't really know what we were doing." She organized a dozen focus groups—

sessions used by advertisers and marketers to understand how potential customers respond to an idea, an image, or a product. In the groups, a professional moderator leads a conversation with six to twelve volunteers chosen by their age, sex, and habits. Researchers behind a one-way mirror study the volunteers' words and demeanor, searching for flickers of deep emotions.

Every Cigarette Is Doing You Damage provoked the smokers in nearly every group. It was "disgusting." "Serious kind of nasty," said one man. Some smokers thought the nastiness was exactly what made the ad powerful. One man called the oozing brain ad "mind-altering. It made me think about quitting. I'm a heavy smoker. I mean, my brain is kind of messed up now." But others said the ad would just make them change the channel. The ad featuring Pam Laffin, who had died after a lung transplant, also hit hard. The one with Ronaldo, with the hole in his throat, hit even harder. Those ads were already on the air, and some smokers recalled Ronaldo too well. "Not the man with the hole," cried one woman when the moderator cued up the ad. "Please don't show me that man because I'm running out of here. . . . He scares me."

The health department team had been excited about *Everybody Loves a Quitter* "because it seemed very positive and kind of an uplifting thing," said Escoffier. "It's a lovely ad," said Beth Kilgore. "It looks like a pharmaceutical ad, it looks like an ad for 'I Can't Believe It's Not Butter,' whatever." In the focus groups, many of the women loved it. "It made me feel happy and hopeful," said one. "It takes away the embarrassment that the other commercials make you feel," said another woman. "The other ones just make you feel guilty." But most of the men were skeptical. "I mean, who needs a hug?"

Advertising agencies measure the dose of TV ads that an audience gets with gross rating points (GRPs), which estimate the percent of the population watching when the ad was shown once, on average. If an agency bought 200 GRPs, it meant that New Yorkers on average saw an ad twice. The health department bought a rapid series of four-week ad blitzes with about 400 GRPs per week, which is about as hefty a dose as political candidates buy during the heat of an election campaign. One woman in a focus group felt as if Ronaldo were everywhere. "I don't want to see him on my TV. Like the one night, I swear, I was turning on my TV, and he came. Hurried it up, changed it. He was on the *next* station. Oh, hell no! I can't take him . . . And if I'm going to quit again, he will be the reason." At around the same time, the New York State health department ran its own antismoking ad campaign, with some ads focusing on the damage from smoking and others emphasizing the dangers of secondhand smoke. Combined, the two health departments hit New Yorkers during 2006 with nearly 11,000 GRPs—on average 110 times—which is about as heavy a blanketing with antismoking ads as anyone had ever done.

Sarah Perl discovered a way to measure the effect of the ads that was less subjective than focus groups. Each ad ended with a plea for smokers to call the city's 311 information line for help quitting. When the Pam Laffin ad hit the air, calls shot up from about 200 per week to over 1,000. Mike Sams drove them up past 1,500. But—something the media team didn't understand at the time—the best was Ronaldo, who propelled nearly 3,000 calls a week.

Most smokers didn't call, though. Frieden wanted to know how the ads affected typical smokers. He had his staff survey 2,000 smokers and more than 400 recent quitters over the telephone. The survey left no doubt that people had felt the ad blitz. Ninety-two percent said they had seen at least one of the antitobacco spots, and half had seen at least three of them. Of those who had seen an ad, 94 percent thought the ad had "said something important" to them, and over half said it had made them want to quit. Ronaldo spurred people to quit the most.

Despite the warm reception it got in the focus group, *Everybody Loves a Quitter* was a dud. Kilgore believes it got lost among all the pharmaceutical ads that it resembled. "We don't have the budgets of those companies," she said, "so we have to look and sound different." "We had that on the air, and the call volume was dying," said Sarah Perl. "But when we put Ronaldo on the air, the call volume spiked back up." It was a lesson they never forgot. Positive messages fail. Done right, scare tactics work. After that, Perl said, "we pretty much abandoned anything that we didn't think was quite hard-hitting."

. . .

When the city passed the Smoke-Free Air Act in 2002, Bloomberg's chief of staff Peter Madonia had worried about political fallout in the next election, November 2005. But the mayor had told him "over and over and over again" that by that time no one would remember the controversy. Bloomberg was right. Within a year of the law's passage, bars and smokers had adapted fully. The mayor told reporters on the anniversary, "I can't go into a bar or restaurant where I don't have people come up to me who work in the restaurant and say, 'I want to give you a kiss, you saved my life.'" The restaurant and bar business was growing. Even former Bronx borough president Fernando "Freddy" Ferrer, a Democratic candidate for mayor, admitted that the smoking ban wouldn't hurt Bloomberg's reelection chances.

In the heated 2005 Democratic primary, Ferrer beat Council Speaker Gifford Miller, Representative Anthony Weiner, and others. In the general election, Bloomberg had so much more money to spend than his opponent that one political scientist called it a "vertical playing field." Ferrer and Bloomberg fought over typical issues—education, jobs, crime, housing, and the city budget—plus Bloomberg's bid to build a stadium on the West Side of Manhattan and host the Olympics. Neither talked about public health. As the election approached, Frieden talked to the mayor's campaign staff, willing to help. By then the communications people saw Frieden as nothing but trouble, the chief nanny in the nanny state. The health commissioner could be most helpful, they told him, by allowing them to "put duct tape over your mouth and put you in a closet."

Bloomberg crushed Ferrer by twenty points. Despite being a white billionaire facing a Hispanic populist, Bloomberg got roughly half of the vote of African Americans and three in ten votes of Hispanics. Two and a half years earlier, after he raised property taxes, his approval ratings had sunk to near 30 percent, and they remained below 50 percent for most of his first term, but shortly after the reelection they soared to 75 percent.

After Bloomberg's victory, Frieden remembers the mayor gathering all his commissioners in City Hall to inspire them for the second term.

He told them that the high approval rating wasn't necessarily a good sign. We have to do big things, he said, things that no one else would do, like passing the Smoke-Free Air Act and building a new aqueduct to bring water from upstate into the city. Big things are controversial. You could argue that if we were really doing a good job, the mayor said, our approval ratings should fall.

And then Ed Skyler, Bloomberg's press guy, called out, "We're counting on you, Tom."

. . .

In June 2006, after Bloomberg gave the speech to the public health law conference that I witnessed, he headed home in his private jet, with Frieden along for the ride. In this rare moment away from the crowds, the mayor was thinking expansively. His foundation had been sprinkling out money for many little things, he told Frieden. But with the foundation, as with his mayoralty, he wanted to do big things. Like eradicate a disease. Could Frieden come up with an idea?

A request like that from a billionaire wasn't something Frieden would let pass. He wanted time to think about it, he said. Bloomberg agreed, then said, "And now I'm going to do a very good imitation of a sixty-four-year-old man taking a nap." And he stretched out and fell asleep.

It didn't take long for Frieden to think up a big thing. Despite the upsetting results from the most recent survey, he figured his antismoking crusade was saving lives by the tens of thousands. The tax increase had worked beautifully. The counter-ads were still unproven, but the calls to the Smokers' Quitline looked promising. And the Smoke-free Air Act was an unqualified success.

The smoke-free law was even spreading. Instead of driving New Yorkers to the suburbs so that they could smoke with their meals, it soon prompted the suburban counties of Westchester, Nassau, and Suffolk to pass their own smoke-free ordinances. Later in 2003 the entire states of New York, Connecticut, and Florida had gone smoke-free. Eight other states followed in 2004 and 2005.

And instead of causing European tourists to avoid New York City, the law was beginning to change Europe. Soon after the city passed it, a delegation from Ireland flew in and met with Christina Chang and others to learn exactly how they had pulled it off. The Irish had been considering a smoking restriction, but after a day of meetings a consulate representative told Chang that his delegation was now determined to push it through. To most people, an Irish pub without smoking was inconceivable. "It's a bad idea," an Irish bartender was quoted as saying. "Cigarettes and alcohol are synonymous, at least in Irish culture." Ireland became the first European country to ban smoking in pubs in 2003, shortly after its leaders visited New York. Then health officials from other European countries contacted Chang to hear the story behind New York's law for themselves.

Frieden thought, what if he were to take the smoke-free law and the rest of the antismoking package to the entire world? Or as he put it later, "What if we had a vaccine that could prevent one in ten deaths worldwide? We already do." Even the world's poorest countries could do it, because indoor smoking bans cost nothing, and cigarette taxes could pay for counter-ads with plenty to spare. All they needed was a political push.

The World Health Organization (WHO) was now calling tobacco the leading cause of death worldwide. It killed nearly twice as many people as AIDS, three times as many as tuberculosis, and five times as many as malaria. But while smoking rates were falling slowly in high-income countries, the tobacco companies were marketing heavily in the world's poorest countries, driving up smoking rates.

Frieden's big idea was to use Bloomberg's money to pay governments (and nonprofit organizations lobbying them) to do what he had done in New York City. "The basic concept was you strengthen the government, you strengthen the civil society, and you put in objective systems to see if it's working . . . and you hold countries accountable." Accountable, that is, for raising cigarette taxes, banning tobacco ads, running counter-ads, passing smoke-free laws, and preventing smuggling. Later he summarized it with the acronym MPOWER, for Monitor (with surveys), Protect (with smoke-free air laws), Offer (help with cessation), Warn (with counter-ads), Enforce (bans on tobacco ads), and Raise (tobacco taxes).

Frieden's proposal was no one-pager. He analyzed data on smoking rates around the world and asked for advice from many experts. Because the city's rules prohibited a city employee from working for someone else during city time, he labored over the proposal on evenings and weekends, mostly alone but sometimes with help from Kelly Henning, another former CDC Epidemic Intelligence Service officer in the health department to whom Frieden often turned for advice and help.

"This was a major, major undertaking," Frieden told me. The final version included the basic strategy, the rollout, milestones, detailed budgets, tables on smoking rates around the world, and even a "risk mitigation" section. He assembled his proposal by hand in black binders of acetate pages at the conference table in his office. It was the kind of secretarial work that would otherwise infuriate Frieden, but he didn't complain. "It was exciting."

"Mr. Mayor," his cover memo began. "As you know, tobacco is now the world's leading killer. Billions of dollars are going to international health but virtually nothing to global tobacco control." His plan would spring from the Framework Convention on Tobacco Control, the first international health treaty negotiated by the WHO. He proposed channeling money to four U.S.-based nonprofits, which in turn would give grants to the WHO, national governments, and advocacy groups. Those organizations would pass the laws, run the ads, and do the surveys to measure the impact. It would all happen in twenty-four months, and it would cost Bloomberg $125 million.

When Frieden presented his case, Bloomberg took it all in. He asked many questions. And then he said he needed to think about it. Even for a billionaire mayor of New York City, this was big.

. . .

In August 2006, in a news conference in NBC Studios, Mike Bloomberg announced that he would donate $125 million over two years to fight smoking in low- and middle-income countries around the world. If the world ignored smoking and current trends continued through the twenty-first century, he said, tobacco would kill one billion people.

Seven in ten of those killed would live in developing countries. Bloomberg's nine-figure pledge to stop that was many times greater than any previous donation for tobacco control anywhere. "I think we've learned some important things about how we convince people to stop smoking," Bloomberg said. "If this kind of progress can be made on a global scale, we can save many millions of lives."

The biggest share of the money would go to five populous countries where about half of the world's smokers lived—China, India, Indonesia, Russia, and Bangladesh—but he would also fund ten medium-size countries like Turkey and Vietnam. Although the program was to start in two months, there were still just two people working on it, Frieden and Kelly Henning, both doing the work only on evenings and weekends.

Frieden penned an article about the initiative in the British medical journal *The Lancet*, with Bloomberg listed as a coauthor, entitled "How to Prevent 100 Million Deaths from Tobacco." That was how many fewer people would die if the world's nations dropped their smoking rates merely from 25 to 20 percent by the year 2020. Frieden wrote, "All nations and populations should be able to achieve this."

. . .

The telephone surveys done in 2006, during and after the antismoking ad blitz, showed that New York City's smoking rate had dropped to 17.5 percent, down 80,000 smokers from the year before and more than overcoming the 2005 uptick. The city now had 240,000 fewer smokers than it had in 2002, for an average of 60,000 quitters per year. The plummeting smoking rate outpaced declines in California and Massachusetts, which were thought to have the best antismoking programs in the country, and the fall was twice as large as that in the United States as a whole.

Looking back, the increase in 2005 might have been a statistical fluke, except for one astonishing finding. In 2006 the group that changed the most was Hispanic men, whose smoking rates plunged from 24.6 to 19.3 percent—meaning that roughly one in five smokers had quit in just that year. It was Ronaldo, Frieden thought. The Hispanic men were responding to Ronaldo. That particular ad, for some reason, was incredibly powerful. Frieden had the results of his "empirical experiment": tough antismoking ads on TV work.

The experience taught his media team other lessons. The women in the focus groups had voted for *Everybody Loves a Quitter* because they *liked* it. But Jeffrey Escoffier and Beth Kilgore realized now that they had asked the wrong question. It didn't matter if smokers liked an ad. The health department wasn't trying to sell yogurt. They were trying to *unsell* smoking. What mattered was whether the ad made smokers squirm.

Smokers had many reasons to brush off health messages. *Everyone dies someday. I'm not as old as the person in that ad. I can quit later if I get sick. Plenty of people smoke and live long lives.* After the 2006 tests, Escoffier told the focus group moderators to stop asking the participants if they liked an ad and instead push hard on "Would this make you think about quitting?" More important, he just watched the smokers in the focus groups to see if they looked shaken. "You have about five seconds of actual response" before they figure out how to deny the message, said Sarah Perl. "If it makes me wince, 'Ahhh, that's horrible', *that's* what you want. . . . That makes you think twice about lighting up."

Escoffier and Perl put *Every Cigarette Is Doing You Damage* back on the air. They imported more ads from Australia, these showing gangrenous toes and operations to unclog arteries filled with fat. And they created a new ad, entitled *Cigarettes Are Eating You Alive*, which showed how "smoking eats away at nearly every vital organ and tissue of the body." It was the toughest ad they had ever seen, highlighting gruesome close-ups of a lung turned black, teeth turned rust-colored, a lip rotting from cancer, and a tennis-ball-size neck tumor. The Australian ads were ugly, but Beth Kilgore thought "we took it to the next level. . . . It was so graphic that I'm shocked that it went on the air." In fact, some television stations refused to run it. When *Cigarettes Are Eating You Alive* did air, Kilgore said, "we saw call volume spike like we've never seen it before."

Escoffier and Perl also reran Ronaldo. In a completely unrelated focus group, they got a crucial insight into why his ad was so powerful. The department had been testing an ad to encourage people to get flu shots. The line meant to scare people into getting vaccinated was that influenza was the third leading cause of death for New Yorkers. The focus group participants "weren't fazed at all," said Escoffier. Instead, they asked, "Okay, what are the first two?" Dying, the team realized, wasn't frightening. "Death is incredibly abstract to people," said Kilgore. The thought of death even offers an appealing peace and tranquility—a break from the struggles of everyday life.

On the other hand, no one wants to suffer. Ronaldo was suffering—not as much as someone with cancer but enough. "He wasn't dying, but he couldn't swim, he had a hole in his throat, he had to use a voice box," said Escoffier. *He couldn't even take a shower without worrying about choking.* And he would continue to suffer like that for a very long time.

The team went with it. They invited Ronaldo to come from Massachusetts to film their own spots. They ran his ads so much that Ronaldo became a minor celebrity in New York City. People stopped him on the street to thank him and ask how he was doing. And Sarah Perl started looking for more spokespeople like him.

5

"Are you sure this will save lives?"

In the early 2000s few people had heard of trans fats, but they did recognize the health crisis of human fat. Between 1978 and 2001 the percent of Americans who were obese doubled. By 2004 two-thirds of Americans were either overweight or obese, which meant that in America it was normal to be unhealthily overweight. The epidemic was afflicting nearly one in ten adults with type 2 diabetes and, by the best estimates, killing about 100,000 people a year. Public health experts across the country held conferences and tried small programs, but no one had a practical solution that matched the enormity of the problem.

But what could they do? The obesity epidemic reflected a collision between biology and economics. Humans have evolved through many more periods of famine than excess, so we are genetically programmed to gobble up any calories within arm's reach. In the last half of the twentieth century—a blink of an eye over human history—food production was industrialized, driving down the price, particularly for foods like chips and soda made from subsidized commodities like corn, wheat, and sugar. Distributors of all types, from fast-food chains to fund-raising school cheerleaders, learned that when they put more food in more places and in larger portions, people bought more, and their profits rose. Every day the food industry tempted people with more food, and every day people grew fatter.

67

Fast-food restaurants were one piece of the problem. The chains had learned that they could drive up profits by charging more for larger portions that cost them virtually nothing more to deliver. They prodded Americans with "Would you like to supersize that combo for only 39 cents?" and usually got a yes in reply. From the 1970s to the 1990s, an average meal of a hamburger, fries, and a soft drink grew by more than 200 calories. Two hundred extra calories a day is enough to cause someone to gain 20 pounds over a year. Across a nation, it is enough to account for the entire obesity epidemic. By the turn of the century, calorie counts at chain restaurants were way off the scale of human needs. At Chili's, some hamburger plates topped 2,000 calories—or more than enough for an average American for the entire day—not even counting the drink.

At the health department, Lynn Silver and her staff struggled with how to rein in fast-food restaurants. One day in 2005 she decided she should just talk to them. She called the head office of McDonald's, who sent its lead nutritionist to the health department. Silver tried out some ideas. Could McDonald's make a healthier children's meal in New York City? Cut down the size of its sugary drinks? Offer healthier "combos," with salad instead of fries, or at least make the default options for the combos healthier? The nutritionist "gave us a long spiel and a slide presentation about how difficult their supply chain was and how it took years to modify," said Silver, and didn't follow up.

Silver's initial strategic plan to prevent chronic diseases included "evaluat[ing] food/calorie labeling on restaurant menus." There were good reasons to think putting calorie counts on restaurant menus might at least slow the galloping epidemic. Most Americans considered themselves overweight, and nearly one-third were trying to lose weight. Even the most dedicated dieters, though, had no way of choosing lower-calorie foods when they ate at restaurants, because they had no idea how many calories the food contained. If they guessed, they were likely far off. In studies, people judging a food item by its appearance or by a description missed the mark by hundreds of calories, usually on the low side. In one study, people on average estimated that a patty melt with fries delivered 800 calories, when it actually packed 1,300. Even professional dietitians grossly underestimated the number of calories in food, guessing that a tuna sandwich had only 370 when in fact it had 700.

Nutrition advocates had been talking about requiring chain restaurants to give customers nutrition information since 1990, when the FDA mandated Nutrition Facts panels on packaged food. Congress had exempted restaurants then because their food often wasn't standardized and because restaurants were traditionally the regulatory turf of state and local health departments. In 2005 anyone could turn over any bag of chips and—with some calculating—learn how many calories were inside, but fast-food customers had to go on a scavenger hunt to find out the number of calories in a Whopper. Chain restaurants did have standardized recipes, so they could calculate calories easily. Most chains put nutrition information on brochures or on websites, and some on densely packed posters on restaurant walls, but others didn't even do that. Only a tiny fraction of customers ever found the numbers.

Posting calorie counts where restaurant customers could easily find them seemed the least the health department should do in the face of the tidal wave of obesity. The counts would justify themselves even if only one in ten customers swapped to a lower-calorie item. And a 10 percent drop in sales of higher-calorie items might prompt the fast-food chains to shrink their portions, or at least slow the arms race of supersizing, which would help even those customers not counting calories.

Since the early 2000s, legislators in at several states, from Maine to Texas, had been trying to pass laws requiring nutrition labeling in chain restaurants. In 2005 Senator Tom Harkin (D-Iowa) introduced a federal bill to do it. But the restaurant chains hated the idea. Their representatives complained their food was far too complicated ("We're not a box of crackers, where every box is the same") and ridiculed the labeling proposals as "the height of absurdity . . . They've been doing it on prepared foods for years, and obesity has increased." With that opposition, the bill stalled.

That same year Brooklyn legislator Felix Ortiz introduced his own nutrition-labeling bill for New York State. The bill appeared in Lynn Silver's inbox. Every year Ortiz introduced a flurry of health-promotion bills that made no progress. Still, his bill made Silver think harder about nutrition labeling. It hit her that the department could instead put the proposal before the Board of Health. Like the trans fat rule, a menu-labeling mandate would be an unusual use of the health code, but it looked legal.

The idea was simple. Translating it into practical rules would be complicated. The nutrition labels had to be prominent enough to hit customers in the face, but because the restaurants would probably sue, the rules could not be unfairly burdensome in the eyes of a judge. The tough decisions, as always, would be where to draw the lines. If the rules require posting of calorie counts at fast-food chains, what about sit-down chains like Ruby Tuesday and coffee shops like Starbucks? If a restaurant had only five city locations, did that count as a chain? Should the department force restaurants to post numbers beyond calories, like the amount of fat, saturated fat, and sodium? Must the restaurants post the counts on the menu board itself, or would a nearby sign do? Could sit-down places list the calorie counts on a separate page of the menu, or must the counts be next to the name of the item? Should Baskin-Robbins post numbers for each flavor or variety? Silver wanted strong requirements—more prominent placement and fewer exceptions. "I pushed pretty hard," she told me. But General Counsel Lopez kept objecting. "And that was good because it raised all the legal obstacles."

In the end the team decided that the location of the nutrition information was crucial. It had to be on the menu board or the menu, right next to the item name and price. The menu board was, they heard later from Burger King, "the single most valued piece of real estate in a Burger King restaurant . . . it is what customers look at, and it is what stimulates their decision to buy." They also decided to apply the rule only to restaurants that already published nutrition information on brochures or websites. By not defining a chain restaurant by its size, they hoped to avoid a court ruling that the Board of Health had exceeded its authority by using economic—rather than health—criteria. And when restaurants complained that they couldn't calculate calories, the health department could counter that the restaurants were already doing just that.

At first Frieden wasn't much interested in nutrition labeling. But as the group got closer to a workable draft of the rule, "I don't know what happened, but then he got *really* interested," said Mary Bassett. He took over the detailed planning. As he did, he made a key decision. The others wanted to require the restaurants to post two numbers: calories and sodium. He thought that was too much clutter, and that what mattered most was obesity. It would be calories only.

· · ·

The press release on trans fats in August 2005 solved the problem that few had ever heard of them. Afterward, stories appeared across the country. They weren't exactly what the health department would have liked. Even though the appeal was voluntary, many papers painted it as a fight. *The New York Times* described it as "the latest salvo in the battle against trans fats." The *New York Post* warned readers that "French fries, chicken nuggets, pizza, cakes, cookies and many other beloved foods may never taste the same again if the city gets its way." The papers treated the health risk as trivial. In a follow-up story, the *Times* health reporter Gina Kolata mocked the scientific rationale, quoting experts who called it merely the "panic du jour." The conservative chatter that followed was about personal choice. People had the right to eat unhealthy food if they wanted to, and the health department had no right to prevent them. Sonia Angell found that argument laughable. When people ordered fries at McDonald's, the workers at the register never asked "Do you want trans fat with that?"

Nine months later, in April 2006, the health department checked to see what the restaurants had done with their request. Inspectors visited another thousand restaurants, looking for partially hydrogenated oils. "From day one we knew the voluntary thing wasn't going to be enough," said Frieden. "But I didn't expect it to have no impact. It had no impact." Half of the restaurants were still using the artificial chemicals. With that utter failure in hand, the team was ready to propose a ban.

As with calorie labeling, caught between technical and legal pressures, the team argued over every word of a trans fat ban. For example, General Counsel Lopez wanted to limit the ban to only "fry oils," which were the easiest sources of trans fats for the restaurants to identify and to change;

but Silver insisted that they also ban trans fats in baked products like pie crusts and hamburger buns. Disagreements like that, she said with a laugh, were "something I was very used to when I worked with lawyers in the past, you know, having fierce debate and back-and-forth."

The pressures strained the team. Silver's stubbornness and controlling style wore on others. One employee said the staff under her felt "terrorized." Mary Bassett had to do shuttle diplomacy between Silver and the lawyers. Bassett told her once, "Lynn, you're like a tugboat. You can pull a heavy load, but you churn up a lot of water."

Silver, on the other hand, believed that she pushed hard for the same reason that Frieden was demanding—because lives were at stake. She thought that criticism of her was in part sexist. A man who stands firm for his beliefs is considered a strong leader, but a woman who does is a bitch. Bassett tried to smooth things over, defending Silver's "tenacity" and trying to "absorb the bad dynamics when smart ambitious people work under pressure."

At the same time, Bassett, like Donna Shelley, was becoming deeply frustrated by Frieden's style. He constantly sought advice from people outside the department, then made decisions himself. Deputies like her were just "operational"—staff to carry out his orders. He routinely bypassed Bassett, contacting Lynn Silver or Sonia Angell directly to get information and issue instructions. "He's a micromanager," she said. "At least he's able to do it. Some people are micromanagers and can't keep up. With Tom it's always a challenge to keep up with him."

As they drew closer to a practical rule on trans fats, Frieden had to get approval from Mayor Bloomberg, which meant first showing the proposal to the deputy mayors in City Hall. They were appalled. "There was this horrible meeting," said Frieden, in which four deputy mayors took him to a room "in some attic of City Hall," and "worked me over." Bloomberg would approve the idea, they told him, and then would be branded a health nut and a nanny-statist. By even proposing a trans fat ban, Frieden wasn't being a team player. Ed Skyler, the former press secretary and now deputy mayor for operations, was "the heavy," but the others chimed in. "I felt like I was being beaten up in an alleyway," said Frieden. He apparently gave as good as he got, though. His staff had created a "one-pager on lives saved," saying that the rule would prevent between 300 and 1,500 deaths a year. If the city didn't ban trans fats, he argued, they—the deputy mayors—were responsible for those needless deaths. It was the line of argument that he made so often that some in City Hall nicknamed him "Dr. Death."

In the end, they compromised: Frieden would delay the Board of Health proposal for three months while he tried a public education campaign. They "wanted me to get a groundswell of 'get rid of our trans fat,'" he later grumbled.

All through the summer of 2006, as the health department staff prepared to present the trans fat ban to the Board of Health, they plotted a public and political campaign similar to that for the Smoke-Free Air Act. They worried not about the Board of Health but about the restaurants, which would fight the rule on whatever battleground they could find an advantage. That could mean the mayor's office, the City Council, the state legislature, the courts, or the press. And the health department staff were trying to blunt the blowback on Bloomberg that the deputy mayors feared.

They honed four messages: *trans fats kill, trans fats are replaceable, no one will miss them,* and *trans fats in food are like lead in paint.* They fine-tuned rebuttals to the charges that would be leveled against them. (The change would be too expensive? A three-pound drum of Creamy Liquid Shortening made of partially hydrogenated vegetable oil cost $17.95, but the same amount of trans-fat-free Canola Liquid Fry Oil was $16.95. The oils would ruin the taste of French fries? Wendy's had tested trans-fat-free oils and people didn't notice the difference.) They drafted handouts for each of the four messages, wrote op-eds for newspapers, and scheduled meetings with editorial boards. They considered how to dramatize their main points. (Could they find a picture of a chemical factory producing trans fats to show how artificial it was? What about an artery clogged with cholesterol?) They tried to undercut the opposition by getting restaurants that were already trans-fat-free to say how easy it was to make the change. They listed politicians to call just before the vote and who should call them. To "soften the ground" with the general public and follow through on Frieden's agreement with the deputy mayors, they distributed 20,000 copies of a brochure on trans fats and ran a few radio ads about their dangers.

As they laid out the schedule, the team decided to offer the Board of Health the calorie-labeling rule at the same time. Lynn Silver said with a laugh, "We figured that way one or the other would get less attention." They then plotted a similar political strategy on the calorie-labeling rule. Far more energy went into the trans fat strategy, though, because in contrast to the scary word *ban*, menu labeling sounded tame.

In September, after the agreed-upon three months of public education, the deputy mayors tried again, hard, to stop the trans fat rule. They wanted more public education, something more intense. And they insisted Frieden not announce any rule in the meantime. "They said, 'Your education program didn't work,'" Frieden told me. "I said, 'I can't educate people about something they don't *care* about.'"

Frieden was deeply upset. How could he call himself the health commissioner if he couldn't take a simple step that would save hundreds of lives a year? He ruminated openly with Chang about resigning. He called others for advice. In the end, he bypassed the deputy mayors by e-mailing Bloomberg directly. "You can imagine how popular that was with them," he said.

The mayor heard out the arguments from his City Hall advisers. And that forced him to choose between his health commissioner and all his top deputies. To get another opinion, he called his friend Al Sommer, the dean of the Johns Hopkins School of Public Health, who was traveling in France. Was this stuff really that bad?

Sommer confirmed that trans fats were unhealthy but said that no one was sure exactly how much. He called Willett's and Frieden's estimates of how many people trans fats were killing "rubbish." They were "extrapolations of extrapolations of extrapolations." If Bloomberg banned trans fats, New Yorkers would head to New Jersey to get French fries. The public bashing wouldn't be worth it, Sommer told the mayor. Don't do it.

Public bashing is my problem, not yours, Bloomberg told Sommer. I just want to be sure the science says it's bad for you.

As Frieden tells the story, Bloomberg's only question back to him was the same as with tobacco: are you sure this will save lives?

Frieden said yes. And Mike Bloomberg told him to go ahead.

• • •

The New York City Board of Health met on September 26, 2006, in a dingy room with a rattling air conditioner, just down the hall from Frieden's office. The board members heard proposals to allow dogs off-leash in designated spots in parks, permit a new screening blood test for tuberculosis, update the safety rules for lifeguards at city beaches, and loosen regulations for altering the sex on the birth certificates of transgendered people. After that Lynn Silver turned on a projector and said she had come to present two proposals to prevent chronic diseases in New York City. "The first involves chemicals that increase the risk of heart disease. Like leaded paint, which is dangerous and replaceable, no one will miss it when it's gone . . . The second will empower consumers to make informed choices."

Following Frieden's script, Silver, Angell, and dietitian Cathy Nonas took the board through slides for each rule—slides that had been refined and debated by the department's lawyers, chronic disease experts, communications staffers, and restaurant inspectors, then edited again, several times, by Frieden himself. At this meeting, the board would vote only on whether to publish the proposed rule for public comment.

When the members voted to do that, though, the national media played it as a major event. The *Times* was the most positive, recognizing Mary Bassett and Lynn Silver's approach to cleaning up the "toxic environment" as something new: "the trans fat plan is the latest in a series of regulations that have placed New York City in the forefront of regulating behavior and products' content in order to benefit public health." Rupert Murdoch's *New York Post* used the proposals to skewer Bloomberg, saying that "a nanny's work is never done" and wondering if restaurants would soon sell only "tofu taters with soy burgers."

Most of the press treated the rule as a control on people rather than on restaurants. CNN polled its viewers with "Do you think the government should police how much trans fat you eat?" Fox News showed a graphic of French fries and a hamburger covered by a red circle with a line through it, headed "FOOD POLICE." "If you go after the French fries and the burgers," their commentator asked, "what's next?" All the network stories implied that trans-fat-free French fries or doughnuts would taste bad. None showed pictures of anyone suffering from heart disease or mentioned how many people died each year from eating trans fats.

The restaurants were irate. They conceded that trans fats were dangerous; they just didn't think that that meant they should stop feeding them to their customers. Like the Smoke-Free Air Act, the rule would damage an industry and kill jobs. Applebee's said that forcing it to use only trans-fat-free products would "have a stifling effect on our industry by limiting the menu choices of New Yorkers," which would mean "people will likely seek restaurant experiences outside the City or will stop eating out." Charles Hunt of the New York State Restaurant Association said the ban would hurt small ethnic restaurant owners, those who make "cannoli, éclairs, egg rolls, or fresh-baked cookies." But it was the National Restaurant Association that came up with the most creative argument: since trans-fat-free oils would have a shorter "fry life," the change meant "more frequent deliveries of oil to restaurants, [which would] exacerbate the bane of all businesses, cab drivers, deliver truck drivers, and residents—traffic and congestion." The restaurant association talked openly about suing.

Dunkin' Brands was the most reasonable. The company had been working since 2003 to develop trans-fat-free doughnuts with the same "taste, mouth feel, and texture" of the doughnuts their customers loved. They were willing to make the change but just needed more time to find the right combination of soybean, palm, and cottonseed oils for the deep frying, and other oils for the icing.

In all the shouting about trans fats, as Lynn Silver had hoped, the press mostly ignored the calorie-labeling proposal. But the restaurants' noises about it were nearly as threatening. Calorie labeling, Charles Hunt claimed, was utterly impractical. "Does every conceivable combination of toppings on a medium pepperoni pizza need to be listed?" By applying the rule only to restaurants that already published nutrition information, he said, the health department was lending "credence to the saying that 'no good deed goes unpunished.'" McDonald's claimed to have a study showing that customers didn't want to see calorie counts on the menu board. A local McDonald's franchisee complained that the new information would slow down the line at the cash register, ruining their "quick service concept."

The restaurants were even more incensed that the decision makers were appointed experts whom they couldn't push around. The New York State Restaurant Association wrote in its newsletter, "For the past five years, NYSRA has successfully defeated state legislation to require menu labeling. . . . Unfortunately, since the Board of Health is not a legislative body, it is very difficult to lobby."

The press reported that the restaurants would try to move the game back to where they had the advantage—the City Council. Council member Peter Vallone, Jr., was said to be drafting a trans fats bill that would overrule the Board of Health, and a newspaper reported that McDonald's had hired a former deputy mayor to "go to war" with Frieden. While the council was the lawmaking body for the city, the Board of Health was empowered by the state to make rules regulating health. City Council members eyed the Board of Health with great suspicion. They felt that their having won a popular election gave them sole legitimate authority. If the City Council and the Board of Health passed conflicting rules, no one was certain who would win in court. And no one in the health department wanted to find out.

Despite that risk, on December 6, 2006, after public hearings, public comments, and revisions, the Board of Health unanimously passed the two rules, making New York City the first city or state in America to ban trans fats and the first to require calorie labels on menus. The calorie-labeling requirement would take effect March 1, 2007. The trans fat ban would start July 1, 2007, for oils, shortening, and margarine, and—in a bow to Dunkin' Donuts—twelve months after that for deep-fried "yeast doughs and cake batters."

After the years of painstaking work, it was a victory to savor. Before the next team meeting, Frieden sent his driver with fifty dollars to an artisanal doughnut shop that already used trans-fat-free oils. He passed the doughnuts around in a quiet celebration. Years later everyone on the team remembered the meeting, not for what anyone said but instead for the warm feeling of success. And for the doughnuts, which Frieden called *"ungodly, incredibly* delicious!"

6

"I just went on a field trip
to Dunkin' Donuts."

My BlackBerry rang early on a Saturday morning in July 2007. It was Tom Frieden. I didn't know him well yet, but I could tell he was upset. Late in the afternoon the day before, lawyers hired by the New York State Restaurant Association, working for the big chain restaurants, had filed their brief on a lawsuit over calorie labeling. He had read it that night. It was "scary," he told me later. "You'd read their case, and you'd say, 'Oh, we're dead!'" Now he was calling out his troops to counterattack.

I had flown to New York City only a couple of weeks earlier to start work as an adviser to Frieden, without the slightest idea of what I would do. Another public health doctor started in his office the same day I did, and when the three of us met, the health commissioner's first words were "I feel like the cavalry is coming over the hill." There were so many things he had to do, he said, and he had so little time. My first assignment, apparently, was to help defend the department against the restaurants.

The lawsuit had caught everyone at the health department by surprise. They had expected a political and legal brawl over the trans fat ban, but the trans fat war never happened. Frieden later assumed that the restaurants foresaw scandalous headlines. "Why should you be exposed to an artificial toxic chemical that can kill you without your information or your consent? And it turned out that the food industry got that and they didn't say a word." It also turned out that, just as Sonia Angell had predicted, the oil change was easy. Restaurants just started ordering trans-fat-free cooking oils, shortening, and spreads, and the suppliers shipped them. Some restaurants had to change "fry oils" more often or strain them between fryings. Some bakeries' black-and-white cookies spread too much in the oven, so bakers had to add more flour. Cake icing made with certain brands of trans-fat-free "butter cream" came out looking ivory instead of a bright white or separated overnight, so some bakeries had to change brands. But that was as bad as it got. Because the restaurants had insisted that finding supplies and changing recipes would cripple them, the health department—with money from the American Heart Association—set up a phone Trans Fat Help Center. But in a city with more than 20,000 restaurants, it was getting all of ten calls a week.

And restaurant customers were oblivious to the change. Not a peep about French fries tasting burned or pie crusts not flaking right. No one drove to Jersey to get trans fats. No damage to the industry, no losses of jobs. "The hot air that had been circulated turned out to be just hot air," said Lynn Silver. There was "a huge amount of fuss, but at the end of the day, the cannolis and the knishes were still there."

Instead, the restaurants grew more agitated about the calorie counts. They had many criticisms. Health advocates or greedy lawyers would sue them over inaccurate counts. The restaurants couldn't possibly post numbers for all the menu options. The cost would break them. One franchise chain argued that because its restaurants were independently owned, it couldn't force them to comply. The restaurants' lawyers started appearing at the health department, pitching alternatives. Wendy's wanted to put calorie counts on posters on the wall, McDonald's on counter mats, and Dunkin' Donuts on stanchions.

Dunkin' Donuts even brought in a mock-up of its sign. Anna Caffarelli, an assistant to Frieden, was thrilled to see the calorie counts in big letters. "I remember kind of waving it in front of Tom's face, and he was like 'it's great.'" She excitedly brought the sign to Lynn Silver, who stopped her cold. If we let them do this, Silver told Caffarelli, it's what all nutrition labeling will be like, with numbers anywhere but the menu board. It *has* to be on the menu board itself, right next to the item name or price. The health department rejected all the restaurants' alternatives.

Two weeks before the rule was to go into effect, the restaurants sued. Those of us within the health department could only guess at their motives. They must have believed the calorie labels would hurt their sales year after year. Maybe with prominent calorie labels, customers would decline to supersize. That possibility excited Frieden and his staff and made everyone determined to win.

The health department lawyer handling the case was Tom Merrill, whom Frieden had just hired from the city law department to replace retiring general counsel Wilfredo Lopez. Unlike most people in the health department, who dressed like graduate students and spoke in numbers, Merrill dressed in business suits and spoke in Latin legal terms. He had a gentle, lighthearted manner, but from his background prosecuting murders in the district attorney's office, he knew how to fight.

When Merrill arrived, he was immediately overwhelmed. At the law department, he was accustomed to researching legal questions for days or weeks, but now people were constantly firing e-mails at him, on exotic pets or HIV testing or restaurant inspections, expecting answers within hours. He was particularly shocked by Frieden's pace. "You send the guy a legal brief and he's read it the next day," he told me. "I was like, 'Oh my god, how does he do this? . . . What is he, Superman or something?'"

The restaurant chains' lawyers argued that the city was preempted from requiring restaurants to post calorie counts by a the federal Nutritional Labeling and Education Act (NLEA), which required the Nutrition Facts panels on packaged food. The legal principle of preemption exasperated everyone at the health department. Corporations usually have much more sway over the federal government than the state government (and more over the state than the city), so corporations enjoy federal laws that wipe out entire areas of possible regulation for states or cities. They could hijack even a well-intentioned federal law like the NLEA to block further progress on nutrition nationwide. With Bloomberg as mayor, the health department could accomplish great things, but not if the department was checked at every turn by the feds.

Although the NLEA let states and cities regulate food in restaurants, it reserved for the FDA the power to regulate "nutrient content claims." No restaurant could write on a menu "Low in fat!"—which qualified as a "claim"—without meeting FDA specifications. The restaurants' legal argument was that a number like "100 calories" on a menu board qualified as a "nutrient content claim" that only the FDA could require.

At a distance, the argument was nonsense. Congress had let states and cities decide what nutrition information restaurants had to disclose. If cities couldn't require restaurants to post calorie counts, then what could they do? But the FDA regulations on the law were hopelessly tangled, and the more confusing they were, the more opportunities the restaurants' lawyers had to exploit them. Frieden, rather than leave the arguing to Merrill, dove into the legal morass. He later called the case "one of if not the most interesting things I saw from my time there."

. . .

Two months and many legal filings later, Frieden gathered Mary Bassett, Lynn Silver, Tom Merrill, and the rest of his nutrition team around the conference table in his office. The mood was grim and tense. The city had lost, its rule preempted by the NLEA. But in his opinion, the judge had enforced the preemption specifically because the Board of Health had applied the rule only to restaurants that already offered nutritional information voluntarily. The provision that Wilfredo Lopez had put in the rule to avoid losing a lawsuit had done just the opposite. For reasons that I still don't understand, the judge had decided that a rule tied to the voluntary act of providing nutritional information on a website made that information a "claim." On the other hand, the judge suggested that he would allow a revised rule that required the posting of calorie information by all restaurants, or by chains of a certain specified size.

With that offer from the judge, Tom Merrill called the ruling "the best loss I've ever had." But Frieden recognized that even if his team rewrote the rule in a way that the judge said would be legal, the health department might lose on other grounds. They would revise the rule, he told his staff, in time for the next Board of Health meeting in a month. And in doing so, they would rethink every single decision they had made in hammering out the original. When I later asked him why he didn't just fix the one flaw, he said, "Because we were the first people to do it. We better get it right." He told his team, "We want to go with things that can withstand a full frontal assault by the food industry."

The rule was only about half a page long, but in the meeting Frieden listed sixteen decisions that they would rethink. The restaurant industry "had tipped their hands on how they were going to get around this in every way," he said to me later. "It's like parenting a teenager. You have to be really clear with the rules."

Frieden drilled his team closely. Every word of the rule carried both legal landmines and loopholes that the restaurants could exploit. The group took on a bit of paranoia. What exactly did they mean by a "chain," a "restaurant," a "food item," or even "for sale"? How should they define a menu board? Some chains had posters with photos with items on the wall. Should those count? Should they require calorie counts for temporary "specials"? Was a combo meal an "item" deserving a single calorie count, or a group of items, for which the restaurants had to list calories for each? "Like people can add in this country," Frieden carped at one meeting.

Should restaurants have to list the calorie counts for salad dressing? Dressings packed many hidden calories, and Lynn Silver wanted to warn people about them. "But we want people to eat *more* salad," said Frieden. "A little ranch dressing makes the medicine go down." But people would be tricked into thinking they were eating healthily, she complained. "Fooling people into eating salad isn't the end of the world," he said.

Item tags were especially frustrating. Boston Market was a chain that was laid out like a cafeteria. It didn't have a full menu board; it had tags on each food tray with the name of the food. Should the rule require calorie counts on every item tag? If it did, then what about Dunkin' Donuts, which had a menu board with prices for categories of items ("doughnuts $1.49 ea., $7.50 dozen") but item tags on the individual doughnuts (glazed, plain, chocolate), each of which had a different calorie count? If the health department demanded calorie labels in both places, would a judge kill the rule as "overly broad"? And if they didn't, would the restaurants drop their menus entirely and just label everything as an item tag? The discussion ran in circles. At one point Frieden gave up. "This one's hard. Let's go to the other ones on the list," he said, and then, looking at his sheet, caught himself. "Ugh, they're all hard."

A few days later I was in the hallway near Frieden's office and heard him call my name. He was racing down the hallway and was short of breath because he had just come up four flights of stairs. "I just went on a field trip to Dunkin' Donuts," he huffed. He described its layout. Maybe he just had to force calorie counts on item tags, he said.

In one meeting, with nothing particular to set him off, the commissioner boiled over. "It's a sham," he fumed. When they put counts on brochures and websites, "they say they're giving this information out, but they know no one is seeing it. It's a sham. I want to say it's a sham. Why can't I say it's a sham?" he demanded, looking around the conference table. His staff was silent and avoided eye contact.

Meanwhile, the restaurant calorie-labeling idea was swirling around the country. The health board in Seattle was poised to pass its own calorie-labeling ordinance. The California legislature had managed to overcome the restaurant lobby and pass a labeling law, but Governor Arnold Schwarzenegger had vetoed it. At one meeting Frieden joked about press questions he might get. "Mike [Bloomberg] and Arnold are friends. They are going to ask if Arnold vetoed this why did Mike allow it? I'm going to say because Mike is stronger."

. . .

In mid-November the television news show *60 Minutes* ran a piece on New York City's calorie-labeling battle. Correspondent Lesley Stahl said to Tom Frieden on camera, "The restaurants do not want to do this."

"They hate it," he said.

She grilled a spokesman for Wendy's. "Aren't you truly afraid that, by listing the calories, you're going to lose money?" she asked him.

"Absolutely not," the spokesman said. "If we were afraid to provide the information, why would we voluntarily provide it?"

The piece then cut back to Frieden saying, "What restaurants are doing now is a sham. They're putting information on websites, and they know perfectly well that very few people see it there."

"The colonel, the king, and the clown," Stahl said, were fighting the health department with "lawyers and lobbyists." But they were "up against a formidable foe, because Frieden has a record of making big industry bend to his will. He's the one who forced smoking out of city bars and artery-clogging trans fats out of city restaurants. Both those bans spread nationwide, which is also happening with his new crusade."

In January 2008 the Board of Health adopted the revised calorie-labeling rule. Eight days later, the New York State Restaurant Association filed suit again.

· · ·

A day after the restaurants filed the second lawsuit, in the vaulted chamber of the New York City Council, the consumer affairs committee hosted a surprisingly heated hearing on an entirely different food initiative. The bill they were considering was meant to put pushcarts selling fruits and vegetables in the city's poorer neighborhoods.

The idea grew out of conversations inside and outside the health department. Mary Bassett and Lynn Silver wanted to help New Yorkers eat more fresh fruits and vegetables. Almost no one in New York City ate the recommended five servings a day, but people in poor neighborhoods ate even fewer. Supermarkets had mostly abandoned those neighborhoods, preferring the suburbs where the land was cheap, giant delivery trucks could maneuver, and customers had more money. That left poorer neighborhoods as "food deserts." A health department survey found that in East Harlem, only a quarter of bodegas sold apples, oranges, and bananas, and only 4 percent sold leafy green vegetables. In the early 2000s, researchers started publishing studies showing that people living farther from supermarkets were more likely to have unhealthy diets and to be overweight. The relationship was surprisingly strong. One group of researchers, analyzing data from over 10,000 people in four states, found that people with supermarkets in their census tracts were 17 percent less likely to be obese, even after taking into account their income, education, and physical activity.

The rising national worry about obesity and the trend toward "natural" foods merged around an activist agenda to put more fruits and vegetables in poor neighborhoods. The city established a position for a food policy coordinator, under Deputy Mayor Linda Gibbs, to do just that. Gibbs had been the commissioner of the Department of Homeless Services in the early Bloomberg years, and the mayor promoted her to be deputy mayor for health and human services—between Frieden and Bloomberg on the organizational chart—for the second term. Gibbs, a small, energetic woman with stylishly white hair, had been in city government for years, mostly in social service agencies and believed in providing one-to-one services, but as deputy mayor she took a liking to public health. At first, she didn't see food policy as city government's job, but later she pushed ideas like zoning rule changes that helped small supermarkets locate in poor neighborhoods. The health department had staff encouraging bodegas in poor neighborhoods to sell more produce, but the stores weren't very interested. Managers complained that their customers just didn't buy fresh produce, so it rotted on the shelves. Under the food policy coordinator, New York City began to offer financial incentives for supermarkets willing to open stores in poor neighborhoods, but that would take years to make a difference. Hearing all this, Elliott Marcus, who oversaw the health department's restaurant inspectors, had come up with the idea of Green Carts.

His inspectors enforced the city's laws on food carts selling on sidewalks. Because street vendors engendered strong but varied opinions, the City Council had put a cap of 4,100 on the number of food cart permits that the health department could issue. Most peddlers sold unhealthy food, like hot dogs, pretzels, sodas, and grilled meat, and they fought over street locations with heavy foot traffic like those in Manhattan's business districts or in front of museums. Many more people wanted food cart permits than the cap allowed, so Elliott Marcus's staff kept a waiting list for permits with about 2,500 names. Marcus's idea was to raise the cap on permits but allow the new carts to sell only fresh fruits and vegetables in poor neighborhoods. If people on the waiting list wanted permits that badly, they would agree. Then without the city having to fund anything, fresh produce would appear on the streets in the South Bronx and central Brooklyn. Poor people would be able to buy apples, avocados, and lettuce as easily as rich people did. Frieden estimated that if the city added 1,500 of these Green Carts, at least 100,000 New Yorkers would eat more fruits and vegetables, which would save about a hundred lives a year. As a bonus, the Green Carts might give hundreds of people a way to make a living.

The food policy coordinator presented the idea to a philanthropist interested in food, Laurie Tisch. She agreed to give the city $1.5 million to outfit the proposed Green Carts with distinctive umbrellas and to train the vendors, many of whom would likely be immigrants speaking little English. Speaker Christine Quinn liked the idea immediately and took on the job of getting the council to raise the cap on permits. Who could be against helping poor people buy fresh veggies?

Quinn soon found out. First, members argued over where to draw the lines: what counted as a food desert deserving Green Carts? Some council members hated food carts; they opposed the bill because they were certain the carts would illegally drift into their districts. Quinn's staff and the health department haggled over maps, definitions, and enforcement rules, trying to ease fears and win votes.

And then the real opposition came out: the supermarkets, the bodegas, and brick-and-mortar green markets, which had earned friends on the City Council by donating to election campaigns. They saw the Green Carts as unfair competition, stores on wheels that didn't have to pay rent and utilities. "And that opposition was *working*," said Quinn.

At the hearing, bodega owners and supermarket owners insisted that if stores weren't stocking fruits and vegetables, it was because people nearby didn't want to buy them. One supermarket owner said that near his store "there are at least 20 food competitors. There is not one single bookstore, and all the schools are overcrowded. Education is a problem. Not food."

It got worse. "The Green Carts, in a way that I did not anticipate, had a racial component to them," said Quinn. Latinos owned many of the city's bodegas, and Asians the brick-and-mortar green markets. Latino council member Hiram Monserrate "would get tons of bodega money and just be a pain in the ass," said Quinn. Chinese-American council member John Liu, who like Quinn had mayoral aspirations, became the defender of the Asian green markets. "Where do we have an example where increasing supply actually increases demand?" Liu was quoted as saying in the *Times*. "That is backward voodoo economics." At the hearing, one Korean green market owner said, "So, fruit vendor eventually flowing down to the street making congestion, will take money, black and white, from store. It's not competition. It's cannibalizing."

Days before the vote, Liu led a protest demonstration by one hundred Korean American business owners on the steps of City Hall. Quinn wasn't sure she had the votes to pass the bill. "It was harder than smoking," she said later. She twisted arms and traded favors. To capture a few votes, she and the Bloomberg team dropped the number of carts in the bill from 1,500 to 1,000 and cut down the neighborhoods in which they would sell.

The backroom maneuvering worked. In late February 2008 the council approved the bill. Within a few months, in areas where 15 percent or more of people on the health department's phone surveys had said they ate no fruits and vegetables at all, entrepreneurs would be allowed to sell whole fruits and vegetables on the sidewalk. No one at the health department knew, though, how many of the people on the permit waiting list would actually be willing to sell avocados in East Harlem. Maybe they all wanted only to sell hot dogs in Times Square.

. . .

Several of us in the health department waited anxiously to hear the judge's verdict in the calorie-labeling case. The revised rule was set to take effect on March 31, 2008, but that month passed without a word. Then on April 16 I heard a rumor that, rather than waiting for the judge's ruling, Starbucks had put up menu boards with calorie counts on them. It was a glorious day in New York City, with a brilliant blue sky and the fresh warmth of spring. I thought I would walk to a Starbucks to see for myself, but first I was scheduled to see the health department unveil a new antismoking campaign.

The city's 311 call center was an open room the size of an airplane hangar, filled with a warren of cubicles, over which hung a giant screen showing constantly updated numbers on how many callers were waiting and for how long. That day the operators, headsets over their ears, were distracted by many television cameras and reporters clustered around a podium, behind which stood Frieden. "Dying young versus not dying young doesn't motivate smokers," Frieden told the pack of reporters. "What Ronaldo shows us is that suffering and being disfigured motivates smokers." Sitting next to Frieden was the health department's new star, about to appear in the department's first homegrown testimonial ad.

Marie was in her fifties, with olive skin and a tough New York accent. Beth Kilgore, the sociologist, had met her when she was doing follow-up surveys of smokers who had requested nicotine patches during the giveaway program. Marie told her a story that was as initially bewildering to Kilgore as it was tragic. Doctors had amputated the tips of her fingers and many of her toes because of smoking, Marie said. She suffered from Buerger's disease, a rare consequence of smoking that causes chronic inflammation of small arteries. The arteries clot off, suffocating tissue like fingers and toes that they supply. After years with the disease, the nicotine patches she got from the health department helped Marie finally quit, but by then she had had twenty-odd amputations.

Beth Kilgore had been looking for smokers who could do a Ronaldo-like testimonial ad. She thought Marie's story was moving and tentatively approached her. Marie bravely agreed to go on camera. It had taken Jeffrey Escoffier three rounds of video shoots, but the team finally had ads they thought would work.

Now Marie sat at the launch press conference next to Commissioner Frieden. "I was in so much pain I was taking 200 mg a day of morphine," she told the reporters. "My doctors were afraid to give me any more." Frieden cued up the ads. They had been shot with dim lighting, with close-ups of Marie's face and her hands. In the ads, Marie told her story bluntly, without emotion. Interspersed with her words were photos of the surgical instruments that the doctors had used to cut through her bones, with background sound effects evoking bones being crushed and labored Darth Vader–like breathing. Marie said flatly in one, "At one point I wasn't even living. I was just alive." Beside her at the press conference, propped among the cubicles, were posters that were appearing that day in subway stations around New York. Marie was holding up her hands, with several fingers missing or partially missing. "I chose to smoke," the posters read. "This is what it cost me."

Frieden led the press conference, but the reporters were drawn to Marie, hounding her despite the press officer's repeated call of "Last question!" Then a photographer asked Marie to hold up her two hands in front of her face. She did, and the photographers snapped pictures and the video cameras blinked on.

I left the press conference with a reporter who was working on a profile of Frieden. On the walk back, we went into a Starbucks. The menu board now had numbers to the right of the options. Next to the 16-ounce iced Caffe Mocha drink listing was the number 200, and next to the flavored latte 250. The reporter stopped a man holding a blended coffee drink that weighed in at 200 calories. She asked him if he had noticed how many calories it had.

"Yeah," he told her dejectedly.

"What did you think?" she asked.

"I was appalled," he said.

"But you bought it anyway?" she asked.

"Yeah."

She asked him if he would buy something lower in calories in the future. "Probably," he said.

And then we crossed the street to the health department, and I headed to Mary Bassett's office. Just as we arrived, I heard Bassett shriek, "We won!" The judge had upheld the calorie-labeling rule. Those numbers would soon appear in thousands of outlets across New York City's five boroughs.

7

"Now, for the first time ever, she could see for herself."

In February 2008, Tom Frieden and Farzad Mostashari brought Mayor Bloomberg to a cramped doctor's office in a poor Spanish-speaking neighborhood in the South Bronx and invited the press. The doctor was an animated man named Sumir Sahgal who, unlike many doctors, made house calls. Now the mayor and the health commissioner were with him to demonstrate, after years of effort, Frieden's attempt to transform medical care in America.

It was software, a computer program that wouldn't just help doctors avoid losing medical charts and bill insurance companies. It would help Dr. Sahgal do what he cared deeply about—keep his patients healthy. Once doctors across the city had it, Frieden hoped, the software would extend the lives of millions.

The idea germinated in the summer of 2003, when Frieden read a study, published in *The New England Journal of Medicine*, that showed just how bad medical care in America really was. A group of researchers studying 6,700 medical records found that patients got recommended services at doctor visits only about half of the time. Low-quality medical care posed "serious threats to the health of the American public," the authors wrote. The U.S. medical care system was, in Mostashari's words, "leaving tens of thousands of lives on the table."

The article bothered Frieden more than it did many in the world of public health. Later Mostashari told me that there was "a little bit of snobbishness in public health circles" about the limits of medical care. In the late 1970s, British doctor Thomas McKeown, in *The Role of Medicine: Dream, Mirage, or Nemesis,* had shown that the great improvements in health that occurred since the late 1800s had had nothing to do with medicine. The epidemics of infectious diseases had dried up with better plumbing and housing; McKeown attributed the rest of the gains to improved nutrition. Some public health people, including me, had written that even in the year 2000 medical care didn't affect life spans much. Medical care typically treats people when they are already sick, we argued, when it is usually too late. It should be called "sick care" instead of "health care." When we get sick, every one of us wants help from a good doctor. But if we hope to live longer, healthier lives, we have to prevent disease, not just treat it. That is what public health is about.

Frieden, on the other hand, was convinced that doctors could save lives by preventing disease on a grand scale—not with coronary bypass surgery or cancer drugs but with simple actions like counseling smokers to quit and treating people with high blood pressure, high blood cholesterol, and diabetes. The problem with medical care wasn't that doctors didn't take those simple preventive steps. It was that they were so unreliable. The key to saving lives through medical care was consistency. Preventing disease with medical care wasn't a technical challenge; it was a quality improvement problem.

Frieden had pressed both Mary Bassett and Lynn Silver when he hired them: how could the health department get doctors to do a better job treating high blood pressure and counseling smokers? The two were more interested in promoting healthy behaviors and creating healthy environments than in improving medical care, but they were willing to try.

In the summer of 2004, they attempted a personal touch. Doctors are accustomed to "detail men" (and women) from drug companies appearing in their offices and delivering drug samples, brochures, and trinkets bearing the drug names. It is a horrible way for doctors to keep up with advances in medicine, because the drug companies are driving profits, not health, but it works; after detail men make the rounds, doctors prescribe more of their drugs. So Frieden, Bassett, and Silver tried "public health detailing"—sending into those same doctors' offices health department workers. In the first wave of public health detailing, the staff passed out pamphlets on how to treat smoking and preprinted prescriptions for nicotine patches.

Over two months, the workers visited 150 doctors' offices in the city's poorest neighborhoods. It didn't work. Only a third of the doctors claimed to be asking their patients if they smoked, and the others didn't sound likely to start. Frieden realized that he was actually stuck with not one but two linked problems: doctors weren't doing the simple preventive actions consistently, and no one—not Frieden, and not the doctors themselves—was able to measure any progress they might make.

Mostashari saw the problem from the point of view of doctors. They didn't want to practice bad medical care—they were just pressed to do many things that felt urgent, and they were distracted. One day while visiting a community health center, he spotted a way to help. The center used computer software that reminded doctors to offer flu shots to patients over sixty-five. When the center turned on the reminder, the percent of seniors vaccinated jumped from about 5 percent to over 40 percent. At that time, fewer than one in five doctors in outpatient clinics in the United States used electronic medical record software, compared to more than half in the United Kingdom and 90 percent in Sweden. And the software they were using mainly just re-created paper systems for the computer screen; they weren't "smart" systems that could help doctors make medical decisions.

Mostashari wondered if digital technology could fix the quality improvement problem. "I thought there was something there," he recalled, "but I didn't have the time to figure out what." He proposed to Frieden that he take a six-month "sabbatical" to think about how software could help doctors prevent disease, especially for the city's poorest patients. The civil service manual had no rule for sabbaticals, but Frieden agreed to let him do it anyway. Nothing he had tried with doctors was working, he told Mostashari. Figure this out.

. . .

Nearly a year later Frieden came up with his own idea. It was in late October 2005, in the heat of Bloomberg's second mayoral campaign, with the election just a couple of weeks away. "It suddenly hit me," he told me later, "that election season is when you get money." The mayor was making campaign promises that would require funding in the second term. The health commissioner wanted to add a pledge by Bloomberg to transform medical care.

Farzad Mostashari was making progress. He thought he saw a way for the health department to offer doctors software with features that both reminded doctors to provide the kind of preventive services that saved many lives, and helped them do so. "The way I looked at this," he told me later, was "how do we have Tom Frieden at the shoulder of every doctor in New York?"

That Friday night in October, Frieden called Mostashari and told him he was going to ask for money to do it. The two worked furiously through the weekend on a plan. They made spreadsheets on "how much *exactly* is it going to cost, and *exactly* how long, for *exactly* how many doctors," said Mostashari, when in fact they had no idea what it would cost. They settled on a plan to get a thousand doctors in the city's poorest neighborhoods to use a new "prevention-oriented electronic health record" by the end of 2008. Frieden hoped to sell the idea, based on his boss's background selling computer terminals to Wall Street, as "the Bloomberg in health." They landed on a request for $27 million to cover both the software and the staff to help doctors trade their paper charts for it. By improving medical care, Frieden claimed wildly, it would save $100 million in health care costs.

On Monday morning, Bloomberg made the promise. The message, Frieden later said, was that "it was really exciting, and it was gonna be high tech, and it was for poor people, it would save lives, it would improve medical care, and it would reduce medical costs." In the frenzy of the last days of the campaign, with fanciful promises and dubious charges flying back and forth by the hour, the newspapers all but ignored the idea. But after the election, Frieden got his $27 million for what they called the Primary Care Information Project.

A small company called eClinicalWorks beat out much bigger competitors for the contract. Mostashari and his team spent the next ten months developing the software with them. The software would be smart, and it would think like people in public health. It would remind a doctor based on a patient's characteristics—like age, blood pressure, and presence of diabetes—what sort of tests or treatment each patient should get to save the most lives citywide. In tech jargon, it was a "clinical decision support system," but to Mostashari, it was Frieden hovering at the doctor's shoulder.

The final version of the software had forty reminders, including counseling smokers to quit, treating high blood pressure, screening for depression, testing for HIV infection, and giving flu shots. The software also could easily create "registries," or lists of patients with a specific chronic health problem (like diabetes or hypertension) who needed checkups. And it automatically calculated measures of the quality of care, like the percent of patients with diabetes whose A1C level the doctor had tested within six months, so that doctors could measure their progress across their entire practice.

And now in February 2008, Mayor Bloomberg arrived at a doctor's office in a converted house in the state's poorest borough to demonstrate these smart features to the world. "Of course, the thing doesn't work!" Mostashari remembered. "It was crashing!" Coders revised it furiously to get Bloomberg through the press conference.

Standing beside a computer loaded with the new software, Bloomberg told reporters he was going to revolutionize medical care. "Think about it," he said. "You get notices for preventive maintenance from your dentist, your pet's veterinarian, even your auto mechanic. Why not your doctor?"

Big clinics could afford electronic medical record software on their own. But in the city's poor neighborhoods, doctors often worked alone or in small group practices without tech support. Bloomberg repeated his campaign pledge to install the software in a thousand doctors' offices by the end of the year and added another promise: that 2,500 doctors serving two million patients would be using it by the end of 2010. Even though the prevention features were still buggy, the mayor advised the rest of the country to follow him. Going national with this software would cost the medical care system $20 billion over five years, he said; that sounded expensive but it was only a tiny fraction of the $2 trillion the country paid for health care annually. "We all deserve treatment when we're sick," he said, "but we'll be far better served by a system that's designed to keep us healthy."

Later, when Frieden visited one doctor's office, he saw the system's potential—and glimpsed a problem that the software wouldn't solve. "A lady came in for [prescription] refills and because her thighs hurt," he told me. The doctor ordinarily would have just dealt with her immediate problem. But the computer's software was rife with reminders. Frieden told the doctor, "She doesn't have Pneumovax, she hasn't had influenza vaccine. You haven't checked her A1C in eighteen months, and the last time you checked, it was twelve. Her blood pressure is out of control, her lipids are probably out of control as well, she's on the wrong medications, she hasn't been HIV-tested, you didn't check her for alcohol or depression. She doesn't smoke—that's good, but you didn't check her for unsafe sex . . ." It took the doctor about an hour to clear all the reminders.

I asked Frieden what the doctor's reaction was. "I think he was in shock. Farzad told me afterward, 'You know, he gets twenty-four dollars for that visit.'"

. . .

Meanwhile the antitobacco program kept winning. The 2007 telephone survey showed smoking rates falling to 16.9 percent, a drop of 60,000 smokers from 2006 and 300,000 smokers from 2002. By Frieden's simple one-third estimate, the decline since 2002 would save 100,000 lives.

The cigarette tax had worked so well that the tobacco team wanted to raise it again. Frieden proposed a fifty-cent increase in the city tax. Antitobacco advocates outside the health department, though, bolstered by the state medical society, organized around a $1.50 increase in the state tax, directing much of the money to the Medicaid program to pay for health care. They ran radio and television ads promoting the idea and lobbied legislators. Frieden wrote to Bloomberg, "From an NYC public health perspective, this would be fantastic. It would reduce the number of smokers by nearly 60,000 in NYC (vs. nearly 20,000 with the 50-cent tax we proposed), preventing about 20,000 deaths (vs. about 6,000 with the 50-cent tax)." The campaign worked. With the state running a huge budget deficit and Governor Eliot Spitzer rejecting an increase in the income tax on the rich, the legislature raised the tax another $1.25, bringing the price of a pack of cigarettes in New York City to about $8.50.

The tobacco team kept hitting New Yorkers with tough ads. Ronaldo, the man with a hole in his throat, had another run, as did Marie, the woman who had lost her fingers and toes. The health department also reran its grisly *Cigarettes Are Eating You Alive* ad. Then they tried an Australian ad called *Separation*. In the ad, a mother is holding the hand of her toddler in a bustling train station. The mother then lets go and disappears into the crowd. The camera zooms in on the toddler who now can't find his mother, his face going from confusion to fear to anguished crying. The voiceover says, "If this is how your child feels after losing you for a minute, just imagine if they lost you for life."

The health department was flooded with complaints. How could the director have been so cruel as to make the little boy cry? But an advertising executive on NBC's *Today* show loved the sucker punch of the smoker making his children suffer. Maybe the director had made the kid cry, the ad man said, "but if it saves 20,000 lives for five seconds, I'll take it. . . . Finally, somebody's getting it right."

The 2008 telephone survey showed that smoking rates had dropped another percentage point to 15.8 percent, meaning a decrease of another 50,000 smokers.

• • •

Frieden might have sold his electronic medical record software to Mayor Bloomberg, but Farzad Mostashari still had to sell it to doctors. He hired a team of young eager staff who mailed out pamphlets, attended Medical Society dinners, cold-called doctors, and showed up unannounced in their offices. The doctors were reluctant because the change was traumatic. The switchover meant shutting down their practice for up to two weeks, after which the doctors had to reconfigure nearly every office task, and then the software required more of everyone's time than paper did. The simple task of writing a note or filling out a form suddenly became data entry, and as with all electronic medical records, the software didn't accept data the way many doctors' or nurses' brains worked. Of the doctors who signed up, some later abandoned the system in frustration.

Many of those who made it over the hump didn't like the "clinical decision support system." They found the reminders annoying. There were too many of them. The doctors would rather use that space on their screens for information they found more useful, like a summary of the patient's medical problems. And they sometimes disagreed with the reminders; the internists wanted to change the frequency that certain tests should be done—like every six months instead of every three—and the pediatricians wanted reminders about vaccinations, not smoking and high blood pressure.

But Mostashari was excited by the possibilities after he visited a doctor in Harlem operating a storefront clinic. An older woman, she wasn't comfortable on a computer. It was slowing her down, but she was "soldiering on." It being winter, Mostashari asked her, "What percent of your elderly patients did you give a flu shot to when they came in for a visit?"

She didn't know but guessed about 80 percent.

He asked if she had ever clicked on a tab that produced a list of patients. No, she hadn't.

He clicked on it, and there were all her patients. "Now you can limit it to those who are over sixty-five," he said, and put in the criterion and clicked again. Then he restricted it to those who had received a flu shot. It was only 20 percent.

That can't be right, the doctor said.

"Now, *for the first time ever*, she could see for herself," Mostashari told me. He told her, "Okay, let's look at who has *not* had a flu shot."

The doctor double-clicked on the first patient on the list, to open her progress note. "Yeah, I guess I didn't give her a flu shot," she said, reading her note. "Mmmm, but she was just here for a refill."

She double-clicked on the second patient to open her progress note. "Oh, I'm working on her blood sugars." She clicked on the third one, the fourth one, and the fifth one. After the fifth patient, she accepted it.

"It was that quick," Mostashari told me later. "She accepted that she hadn't given flu shots to eighty percent. Not eighty, not sixty, not fifty, not forty, not thirty!"

The doctor looked a little ashamed. "Can I send them a letter?" she asked.

"Yes you can," he said. "Right here. Just click, and you can send them all a form letter."

Years later he told me, "That was for me the 'aha!' moment, that we can actually get normal docs in that normal storefront who are practicing independently to understand population health."

The doctor's reactions also explained a paradox in medicine. Every doctor believes he or she is delivering excellent medical care, but all the numbers say that medical care in America is abysmal. The discrepancy is that doctors have no idea what they are doing across their entire panel of patients. They remember the difficult diagnoses, the gratifying cures, the tragedies avoided, and the occasional mistakes, but they have a blind spot for the diagnoses, treatments, and counseling opportunities that they miss. Now a computer was filling in the blind spot.

8

"There's no doubt our kids drink way too much soda."

When I first came to the health department in the summer of 2007, Tom Frieden asked me what I thought he should do about obesity. Like Lynn Silver and Mary Bassett, I saw the source as a toxic food environment, especially cheap, calorie-dense, ready-to-eat foods and beverages, offered at arm's reach everywhere from office vending machines to hardware stores. Calorie labels might help some people resist the Bacon Double Cheeseburger at Burger King, but they wouldn't touch the rest of that smorgasbord. I didn't have a simple solution.

Frieden surprised me by responding that he thought the single best action we could take was to put a tax on soda. And with that, he started down a course that would shape the nation's response to the obesity epidemic.

Obesity researchers then were starting to eye sugary drinks with great suspicion. For decades, dietary guidelines had told Americans to cut back on fat. When it came to weight gain, most experts thought, a calorie is a calorie, no matter the source. Because dietary fat has more than twice as many calories per gram as carbohydrates or protein, people should avoid fat. Then in the 1990s, some nutrition experts—watching obesity rates surge despite that advice—started rethinking carbohydrates. During the

101

thirty years of the obesity epidemic, Americans' diets had grown by 200 to 300 calories a day, nearly all from carbs.

In 2002 reporter Gary Taubes stoked a national fad for low-carb diets with an article in *The New York Times Magazine* called "What If It's All Been a Big Fat Lie?" He quoted some scientists who argued that eating carbs floods the bloodstream with sugar, which triggers a sharp release in the hormone insulin. Insulin brings blood sugar down and also tells the body's cells to store fat rather than burning it. After a carb-led surge in blood sugar, the scientists argued, the outpouring of insulin is so great that within about two hours the blood sugar crashes down to below normal levels. That low blood sugar makes people feel hungry, prompting them to eat more. By this line of thinking, a calorie *wasn't* just a calorie. Maybe it was the starchy potatoes in French fries that made you fat, not the grease they were cooked in.

The argument that the blood sugar surge and crash was to blame for obesity wasn't mainstream thinking, but it had some intriguing studies behind it. In one study, when researchers gave a dozen overweight teenagers a carbohydrate lunch that caused a blood sugar surge, later in the afternoon the teens got much hungrier and, compared to a typical day, ate an astonishing 600 more calories.

At around the same time, Dr. Robert Lustig was arguing that sugar is not just another carbohydrate but is uniquely bad—he called it toxic—because it interferes with metabolism in the liver. Cane sugar has two pieces, glucose and fructose. Fructose, Lustig believed, is as damaging to the liver as alcohol. When it hits liver cells, he argued, it sets off a hormonal chain reaction causing chronically high insulin levels that, over years, lead to obesity and diabetes.

Yet another group of researchers were showing that calories in beverages are not nearly as filling as calories in food. A startling example was their study involving jelly beans. The researchers gave fifteen young adults over four-week periods 450 calories of sugar a day in the form of either soda or jelly beans. When the young adults ate the jelly beans, they compensated by eating less of other foods, cutting down their calorie intake by even more than the 450 calories in the jelly beans. But when the people drank the soda, they didn't just fail to compensate—they actually *increased* the calories they ate from food. Studies outside of food labs also started to point a finger of blame at sugar in liquid form. In several studies, including one that tracked more than 50,000 nurses for eight years, people who drank more soda gained more weight.

In the end, it didn't matter much to the health department whether soda leads to weight gain because it delivers unnecessary calories, or because those calories come from carbohydrates, or because those carbohydrates are sugar, or because the sugar is in liquid form. Sugary drinks make people fat.

And that mattered very much, because Americans were guzzling sugary drinks. Over the previous quarter century, per capita sugary drink consumption in the United States had more than doubled, in parallel with the rise in obesity. The average teenager in 2000 drank 300 calories (24 ounces) of sugary drinks a day. Many teens drank twice that. Sugary drinks accounted for 40 percent of the sugar that people ate and between a third and a half of the total increase in calories in Americans' diets over thirty years. Sugary drinks had not caused the entire obesity epidemic, but they looked to be responsible for a big chunk of it.

Lynn Silver had included a soda tax in the long list of ideas in her initial plan for chronic diseases, and within a few months of starting her job in 2004, she further developed the idea in a memo for Frieden. Economists' studies suggested that a 10 percent increase in price should cause a nearly 10 percent fall in soda sales. She proposed two options. The tax could be 2 cents per 12-ounce can, which would only raise money to run an obesity prevention program. Or it could be 2 to 3 cents per ounce, which would roughly double the price of a 2-liter bottle and increase the price of a 20-ounce bottle from $1.25 to $1.65 or $1.85, cutting into sales. At the time, Frieden wasn't ready to fight for a tax, but Silver kept the idea percolating.

In 2006 Silver tried to talk to soda companies, just as she had tried to talk to McDonald's the year before. She called PepsiCo headquarters in nearby Purchase, New York, and was able to get a meeting with the North American president. At the meeting, she and Frieden asked what PepsiCo could do in New York City to accelerate the shift from drinks loaded with sugar to those without it. The two suggested a few marketing ideas for no-calorie drinks, like lower prices, better store placement, and redirecting advertising dollars toward them.

At the time, Pepsi CEO Indra Nooyi was trying to give Pepsi an image as the healthier company. At the meeting, the Pepsi executives talked about their "healthier product" portfolio and agreed to try a pilot program in New York to promote healthier drinks. But they didn't pick up on any of Silver's ideas. "It basically fizzled," Silver recalled later. "We never felt like they were really willing to steer the ship in a different direction." The soda money-making engine clearly had the company trapped. Later, Nooyi had to backtrack from her healthier image to mollify Wall Street investors, who thought that by straying from the core brands of high-calorie soda and chips, she was hurting profits.

In 2007 Mary Bassett invited me to join a group she hoped would come up with ideas for reducing New Yorkers' consumption of sugary drinks and other junk foods. The smoking program inspired three ideas. The cigarette tax had worked, so we revived Silver's soda tax idea, and we also thought about taxes on junk food. TV ads were a success, so we decided to try counter-advertising against soda or junk food. Smoke-free workplaces were winning, but what was the parallel for food? People revolted at the idea of "food-free workplaces," but the group pursued the idea of making workplaces junk-food-free.

One idea didn't get very far, at least not then. Lynn Silver turned to Tom Merrill at the first meeting and asked whether the city could pass a law banning soda bottles bigger than 6 or 8 ounces. For a few seconds, Merrill looked as if he had been hit over the head by a brick. The idea of prohibiting 2-liter bottles, 20-ounce bottles, or even 12-ounce cans of soda throughout the city just felt outrageous. After recovering Merrill asked, "Do you mean legally or politically?" He looked into it anyway and came back with a no.

In the spring of 2008, two things made Frieden think seriously about a soda tax. First, the housing market crash of 2007–8 had crippled Wall Street, the state's main financial engine, slashing tax revenue. Like the cigarette tax, a soda tax would need approval by the state legislature, and the legislature would now be desperate for money. And second, the mayor was nearing the end of his second term, so this looked like the last chance to push big public health ideas. Frieden asked me to estimate what a soda tax would do. I created a model that suggested that a tax of 1 cent per ounce would raise $1.2 billion, cut calorie intake from sugary beverages by 10 percent, and over one year might reduce the number of obese people statewide by 75,000 and prevent 10,000 people from developing diabetes.

In June 2008 Frieden pitched the soda tax to Mayor Bloomberg. First he put up a slide showing the state's projected $8 billion budget gap. "New York State is broke," he said. "This is a good thing for us." Much of that deficit came from soaring Medicaid costs, especially for illnesses related to obesity. Aside from the human suffering that obesity caused—700,000 New Yorkers with diabetes, 2,900 of whom needed amputations and 1,700 of whom died from the condition annually—the epidemic, Frieden explained, was costing city residents more than $4.5 billion a year in medical care. A tax on soda would encourage people to drink less and contribute to reversing the obesity epidemic; it was a tax that no one would be forced to pay because everyone could buy unsweetened beverages or drink water for free. The businessman in Bloomberg understood economics and was proud that his cigarette tax was cutting smoking rates. Getting a soda tax through the state legislature would be very tough, but he was willing to try.

. . .

In the summer of 2008, calorie counts bloomed on menu boards across New York City. Many New Yorkers were stunned. A smallish slice of lemon loaf at Starbucks was listed at 440 calories—nearly one-quarter of a typical woman's daily calorie budget. A Big Mac combination meal—one that *wasn't* supersized—rang up 1,130 calories. A *Times* reporter caught up with a marketing specialist who learned that his Whopper combination meal contained 1,720 calories. The foods offered at sit-down restaurants were even worse: Pizzeria Uno's Individual Chicago Classic pizza was 2,310 calories. One columnist wrote that the new menu boards were like "a poster about herpes at an orgy."

But no one knew how many New Yorkers would actually use those calorie counts or how. In the early days, Kelly Christ, one of Frieden's assistants, wasn't encouraged when she heard a woman waiting in line at Starbucks say with a sweet Southern accent, "Look, y'all. The doughnuts are only four hundred calories. I might could get two." With experiences like that, the health department in 2008 ran ads in subways to ground people. "2000 calories a day is all most adults should eat," the posters read. "Read 'em before you eat 'em."

Rather than depending on customers alone, the health department team was hoping that embarrassed chains might discontinue their 1,500-calorie sandwiches or shrink their 800-calorie snacks. By late summer, Dunkin' Donuts had announced that it would add two egg-white sandwiches below 300 calories. I read in blogs that Starbucks customers had picked clean the lower-calorie pastries by the end of the day, while the high-calorie pastries were still stacked up. Soon Lynn Silver noticed that "mini-scones and teeny chocolate chip cookies" appeared in the Starbucks display cases.

But that was just Starbucks. A few months later I stopped in at a Dunkin' Donuts shop in lower Manhattan and asked the man working the counter whether customers noted the calorie counts. "All the time," he said with a Spanish accent, "every day."

"What do they say about them?" I asked.

"They say, 'Why do they have to have that there?'" He shrugged. "I say it's not up to me, we have to do it. I just work here."

"Do they switch to doughnuts with lower calories?" I asked.

"I don't know about that. . . . But maybe it's a good thing for some of the women."

"Do they leave after seeing how many calories all these doughnuts have?"

"No. They like their doughnuts."

• • •

The idea of creating "junk-food-free workplaces" wasn't entirely new. Mary Bassett and Lynn Silver didn't use that phrase, but the health department had actually been working on them for years. The key step was to write standards that distinguished healthy food from junk.

In 2003 the New York City public school system made its cafeteria food healthier by switching to low-fat milk. Soon afterward it limited sodium and cholesterol and added fruits and vegetables. Then one day Silver spotted a report showing that one in three children in Head Start preschool programs were already overweight. "I thought, 'Wow! This is early!' Waiting until school is too late." New York City's health code already had regulations for child care centers, written during a burst of interest in day care in the 1950s. Silver decided to add rules to help prevent obesity. Her rules banned sugary drinks and limited juice, required low-fat milk, made drinking water readily available, and limited television time. Compared to the fights over trans fats and calorie labeling, enacting the day care standards proved surprisingly easy. Frieden liked the idea, and so did the Board of Health. Very few people complained about the new rules during the public comment period, and the board passed them.

That opened another idea. New York City likes government. Its huge network of agencies provide some 260 million meals and snacks a year through more than 3,000 sites: not just schools but also jails, senior centers, homeless shelters, public hospitals, day care centers, after-school programs, and programs for people with mental illness. When Linda Gibbs's food policy coordinator arrived, he realized that the entire city government could set a healthy example. The coordinator brought together the twelve city agencies that gave out the most food, and over a year and a half of meetings, the health department wrote food standards that were more detailed and extensive than could be found anywhere else.

The agencies disagreed, and it wasn't easy to settle the arguments. The public hospitals had their own nutritionists and resisted citywide rules. (Their doctors liked to write orders for cranberry juice, which has more sugar than Coca-Cola.) The jail system fed more than ten thousand prisoners, who scrutinized their trays. "This is about more than just food," Silver remembers the jail staff saying. "We have to be careful that we don't create a riot. These guys will be really upset if they get one less slice of bread or can't get their Coke." But ultimately the agencies agreed to one set of rules. There were standards for foods that the agencies purchased that banned sugary drinks, and standards for meals served that required two servings of fruits or vegetables at lunch and dinner. The city's contracting agency then wrote the standards into contracts with the nonprofit organizations that ran programs funded by the city. Even group homes for people with mental illness—who tend to die young of diabetes and heart disease—would now serve meals with fruits, vegetables, and whole wheat bread and without soda.

Then Mary Bassett's junk food group, and later the food policy coordinator, trained their sights on vending machines. In the early 2000s health advocates across the country began agitating to banish vending machines from schools. State legislators introduced bills, which the soda companies mostly beat back. In 2006 Bill Clinton—who had never before dabbled in nutrition—swooped in to announce an agreement with the soda industry. The soda companies said they were eliminating full-calorie soda from school vending machines, but the rules left some important loopholes, like allowing high schools to sell so-called sports drinks, and delaying the implementation until 2009.

The New York City health department wanted to go further and ban all sugary drinks from school vending machines. Like schools across the country, New York's were making money from soda vending machines—about $6 million a year citywide—much of which paid for athletics in middle schools. The soda sales were not so big that by themselves they contributed much to obesity, but they amounted to an endorsement that encouraged children to drink sugary drinks everywhere else, too. After plenty of back-and-forth between agencies, during which Lynn Silver "felt like I was the person who was being a stubborn pain in the butt," the schools adopted stricter standards. In schools and other places regularly used by children, vending machines could sell only water, unsweetened low-fat milk, and drinks with fewer than 25 calories per 8 ounces. All bottles had to be labeled with calorie counts, artificial sweeteners were prohibited, and the vending machines themselves couldn't advertise sugary drinks.

If sugary drinks were bad enough to merit their own tax, the health team felt that they didn't belong in other government buildings either. Unlike other cities, New York went on to write vending machine standards for the other government agencies. It proved much harder to take soda out of adult spaces than schools or day care centers. The best the food policy coordinator could manage was to limit sugary drinks in vending machines to two slots and to balance that with more slots of bottled water. But at least the city government now *had* anti-junk-food rules—rules that the health department could shop around to other organizations.

· · ·

By the end of 2008, New York State's plunging tax revenues had ballooned the projected deficit to $15.4 billion, creating the largest budget crisis in the state's history. On December 17 Governor David Paterson, who had succeeded Eliot Spitzer after Spitzer was caught in a prostitution scandal, presented his plan to manage the crisis. "We're going to take some extreme measures," Paterson told the state legislators. He proposed $9 billion in spending cuts, including big whacks in education and a $1 billion cut in payments to hospitals, nursing homes and other medical providers. He also proposed 137 new taxes and fees, one of which he called an "obesity tax"—an 18 percent sales tax on sugary drinks.

Paterson's "obesity tax" was Tom Frieden's soda tax, only mangled by the state's Office of Management and Budget. Frieden had proposed an excise tax, paid by distributors based on the ounces of sugary drinks they shipped to retailers. The state agency had converted it into a special sales tax paid by retailers, who already paid the state's regular sales tax.

The state's version would help with the state's budget crisis, but it nearly ruined the potential health benefits. First, unlike an excise tax, the sales tax would not appear in the price on the bottle or on the grocery shelf but instead would be added at the cash register. Most shoppers buying a basket of groceries would not see how much extra the soda cost them. Second, the cost of soda on a per-ounce basis varied dramatically with the size of the bottle. A 20-ounce bottle of Coke in a vending machine often sold for $1.25—the price of a 2-liter bottle in a grocery store. The per-ounce excise tax proposed by Frieden would have added 20 cents to the 20-ounce bottle but 68 cents to the 2-liter bottle, encouraging people to switch to the smaller sizes. On the other hand, an 18 percent sales tax would add the same 23 cents for the two sizes, which might even inspire consumers to choose *larger* bottles to get the better "deal."

Nonetheless, for the first time ever, a governor had proposed a tax on sugary drinks to combat obesity. It was a new idea—after calorie labeling, the first serious public policy proposal to respond to the epidemic. And the mayor of the nation's largest city—the man who was becoming recognized as the nation's loudest public health advocate—was cheering him on. At Paterson's state of the state address in early 2009, Bloomberg said that "the governor is 100 percent correct . . . obesity is the single largest public health issue in this country that is growing. We have to do something about it." He would work with the legislature on the final shape of a soda tax, "but to sit back and let our kids get themselves into a health situation where they're going to get diabetes and die is not something we can do."

Paterson's proposal stirred up a national conversation about the sugary drinks, obesity, and taxes. Health experts generally loved the sugary drink tax. The big soda companies hated it, which we took as a signal that it would work. A spokesman for the American Beverage Association, the lobby group for Coke, Pepsi, and the other soda companies, promised to fight, calling the tax "purely a money grab that would be paid for by hard-working New York families" and that would damage and industry and kill jobs.

Frieden mobilized his team to do two things at once: support the idea but change it to an excise tax. Gaining the support of the Greater New York Hospital Association (GNYHA) and of the SEIU 1199 union, opponents in wage negotiations, was crucial. The hospitals floated on state Medicaid funding, which Paterson proposed to cut. The GNYHA would lobby hard against the $1 billion cut, but if the sugary drink tax failed, the governor would likely reduce Medicaid even more. The SEIU 1199 union represented health care workers, like nurses' aides, clerks, and maintenance workers at hospitals, nursing homes, and home care agencies. To them, Medicaid cuts meant job losses. At Frieden's urging, the groups issued a joint statement saying they strongly supported the tax, then pivoted to propose changing it to a penny-per-ounce excise tax.

Voters, who never like taxes, weren't enthusiastic. A community organization called the Citizen's Committee for Children found that 52 percent of voters supported "a one-cent-per-ounce tax on all sugar-sweetened beverages—and using a portion of the money to combat obesity in children and adults." But a polling unit at Quinnipiac University, asking the question differently, got a far worse answer. Only 32 percent of voters supported "an 'obesity tax' or 'fat tax' on non-diet sugary soft drinks."

Then Paterson—who struggled in the governor role—undercut himself. Only a few weeks after proposing the tax, at a town hall meeting with college students in Morrisville, he told the "soda addicts" not to worry. "The tax on soda was really a public policy argument," he said. "In other words, it's not something that we necessarily thought we would get." His spokesperson tried to backpedal, saying that "the governor stands firmly behind his soda tax proposal," but the damage was done. Soon the federal government passed a financial stimulus package, sending money to New York, which relieved some of the budget pressure. In budget negotiations with legislators, Paterson abandoned the soda tax.

They say it takes three years to get anything through Albany, I was told. My colleagues at the health department and I consoled one another that we got the idea "out there." Next year or the year after, we would get it passed.

Paterson's proposal certainly succeeded in getting the idea out there. Silver and Frieden's idea channeled a growing national frustration about the obesity epidemic toward a specific, simple solution. Suddenly people around the country were talking about soda taxes. Frieden and Kelly Brownell, a longtime anti-obesity researcher and advocate, wrote a piece in *The New England Journal of Medicine* promoting them. David Leonhardt, an economic columnist for *The New York Times*, wrote a column calling their arguments "fairly compelling." In Washington, congresspeople trying to figure out how to finance Obama's health care reform plan proposed a soda tax. Obama himself, when asked about it, said, "It's an idea we should be exploring. There's no doubt our kids drink way too much soda." Fox News stalwart Sean Hannity attacked it: "We can't live anymore!"

Even Stephen Colbert, in faux-conservative character, ranted against the soda tax, saying those who wanted it would have to pry the can of soda "from my cold, diabetic hands." He ridiculed American Beverage Association president Susan Neely's remark that "soft drinks don't play any role in the obesity epidemic. Soft drinks are just a fun beverage along with a lot of other beverages and foods that we like to eat or drink."

"Yeah, things that are fun are never bad for you," Colbert shouted. "We learned that from unprotected sex!"

9

"In the end, it's just ketchup."

It finally caught up with her. After many years doing everything right, Sylvia Birnbaum (not her real name) learned that she had high blood pressure. Even months later she said, "I'm still in shock."

Sylvia Birnbaum had always protected her health. Her husband, not so much. He smoked a cigarette first thing in the morning and last thing before going to bed, and in between he always seemed to have a cigarette in his mouth. One day when he was on a business trip at age forty-three, he had a heart attack. Unlike Chris Gallin, he never came home.

Afterward Sylvia Birnbaum was even more vigilant. Every workday, instead of taking the elevator to her desk on the third floor, she walked up the stairs. She read food labels and tried to choose healthy food. She ate no-added-sugar cereal for breakfast, salads for lunch, fruit for snacks, and chicken or fish, with a vegetable on the side, for dinner. With that, she stayed thin—120 pounds, five foot three. And for many years she did what almost no one else who doesn't already have high blood pressure does: she avoided salt. She didn't have a saltshaker in her apartment. She ate no-salt cottage cheese, crackers with unsalted tops, and—for an occasional treat— no-salt potato chips. Taking in so little salt, she lost her taste for it, so now if she gets something salty, she doesn't like it.

But one day her doctor said her blood pressure was 140 over 90. Several

*visits and measurements later, her pressure was still high. The doctor told
her she should take a pill every day for the rest of her life to reduce her risk
of a stroke or heart attack.*

*Looking back on it, she realizes that there was plenty of salt that she
hadn't been avoiding. She had a taste for canned butternut squash soup.
Her breakfast cereal had salt in it. The crackers had sodium in the wafers.
And when she went to a restaurant, she had no idea how much salt was in
the food.*

· · ·

By one estimate, hypertension—high blood pressure—kills nearly
400,000 Americans a year by causing heart attacks and strokes. That's the
size of the city of Minneapolis. Almost two-thirds of people over sixty
have the condition. That means hypertension shares with obesity the disturbing combination of being distinctly unhealthy yet so common that
we can only call it normal.

Tom Frieden wanted to nudge doctors to do a better job treating
patients with hypertension. But in early 2005 Lynn Silver came across a
report from a nutrition advocacy group that made her think very differently about the problem.

The report carried the menacing title *Salt: The Forgotten Killer*. For
decades, researchers have eyed sodium, as in sodium chloride, as the
prime suspect for hypertension. Give lab rats extra sodium, and they
get high blood pressure. The same is true for dogs, chickens, rabbits,
baboons, and even our very near cousins, chimpanzees. Put people on
low-salt diets, and within weeks their blood pressure falls. In two isolated
tribes of Solomon Islanders, the one that used seawater for cooking had
higher blood pressure than the one that didn't.

In the 1980s a huge team of researchers carried out a study called
INTERSALT, in which they measured sodium intake and blood pressure in fifty-two strikingly different populations around the world, from
residents of Beijing to the Yanomami Indians of the Amazon jungle. The
populations that consumed more sodium had higher average blood pressures. Among the study's four remote native populations who took in a

fraction of the salt that we do, virtually no one had high blood pressure, even as they got older. The scores of studies on salt fit together to tell a story that people have hypertension today mostly because, over their lifetimes, they eat way too much sodium. High blood pressure isn't an inevitable part of the aging process, then. It is more like a marker for chronic sodium intoxication.

Ever since our ancestors abandoned the oceans for dry land, they have needed to eat salt for their internal biochemistry. But for most of evolutionary history, away from the sea, salt was difficult to find. That's why land animals constantly seek it out, why hunters can attract game with salt licks, and why we humans crave salt. Salt was so scarce in the Paleolithic period that, by the best estimates of archaeologists and nutritionists, our hunter-gatherer forebears took in less than a third of the sodium we do—but about as much as those remote tribes consumed in the 1980s. It is an anomaly in human history that salt is now plentiful and cheap.

Salt now costs far less than spices and other ingredients, so food companies pour salt into processed food to play to our craving. Salt appears in processed foods even where we don't expect it or taste it. Ham and canned soup are full of salt, but so is breakfast cereal and bread. A blueberry muffin has almost twice as much salt as a serving of potato chips. All that salt leaves Americans taking in about 3,500 mg of sodium (about 1½ teaspoons of salt) per day. Fewer than a third of Americans take in below 2,300 mg, and fewer than one in ten take in below 1,500 mg, two recommendations for healthy sodium intake.

If Americans were to take in a little less salt, far fewer of us would have high blood pressure. Changing people's diets has big advantages over treating them with medicine for hypertension. First, it would save many doctors and patients the trouble of making the diagnosis, getting the prescriptions, and swallowing those pills every day for a lifetime. Second, it would make it easier to treat hypertension when it happens anyway. Third, and most important, it would lower the blood pressure even of people in the "high normal" range—much of the entire nation—which would cut their risk of heart attack or stroke also.

Doctors recommend that people with high blood pressure go on a low-salt diet. But cutting salt significantly is nearly impossible, as Sylvia Birnbaum found out, because nearly 80 percent of the sodium that Americans eat comes in packaged and restaurant food. The only way to prevent millions of Americans from developing hypertension is to get food companies and restaurants to stop loading their foods with salt.

That's where it gets complicated. People love the taste of salt itself, and salt enhances other flavors. Take salt out of canned soup, and it tastes like dishwater. But it is possible to reduce sodium in food without making food taste awful. Food companies often use salt or sodium for reasons that have nothing to do with taste, like leavening or food texture. And competing foods made by different companies have wildly different sodium levels, which shows that companies can cut the salt in their recipes sharply without hurting taste. Scientists have shown that when people eat less salt, even for as little as two months, their preference for a salty taste drops. Sylvia Birnbaum saw this. If all companies were to reduce the amount of salt they use gradually, their customers' taste buds would adjust without anyone noticing.

Lynn Silver was always looking for the Holy Grail in public health: actions that have a big health benefit, can reach a lot of people, and are inexpensive. Prohibiting trans fat met those three criteria. Cutting salt in food felt to her like another Holy Grail, a change that no one would notice but that could save many thousands of lives. Finland once had astronomical rates of heart disease. In the 1970s the government started a national campaign against salt, and in 1993 it required manufacturers to post high-salt warning labels on foods that were really loaded. The food companies cut back, salt intake dropped by one-quarter, and deaths from heart disease plummeted.

In this country, the federal government had been trying—feebly, but trying—to cut salt in the food supply for decades. It first asked food companies to reduce sodium in 1969. In 1978 the Center for Science in the Public Interest petitioned the FDA to regulate sodium levels and to require companies to put warning labels on high-sodium foods. Ronald Reagan's FDA wasn't about to create new regulations for food companies, but in 1981 the FDA said it would "encourage" the companies to cut back "where this is safe and feasible." Two years later it called the results "encouraging." But the FDA didn't track salt levels in foods, and a quarter-century later surveys showed that Americans' sodium intake had instead increased.

Silver handed the *Forgotten Killer* report to Sonia Angell and asked her to think what the New York City health department could do. How could a city agency change America's food industry when the federal government had failed for so long?

Their authority wasn't clear. State and local health departments in the United States generally don't regulate the content of food. The FDA does that, and federal law preempts state and local laws. Still, "we had this lovely example of an effective model" in trans fats, said Angell. "There was no reason we couldn't do it ourselves."

But salt proved much more complicated than trans fats. Because humans need salt, the health department couldn't ban it. Angell wanted only to reduce it. But to what level, and in what foods? Salt showed up in thousands of foods, from sausage to cookies. No one category of food was a standout culprit. The top five—bread, cheese, ham, salad dressings, and sweet baked snacks—together accounted for only about 25 percent of Americans' salt intake. And lowering the salt levels in some foods would be tough. Ham was laden with salt less for taste than as a preservative. "You're never going to outlaw a pickle," an expert told me. Setting a maximum level for salt that accommodated ham or pickles would be like setting a national speed limit at 150 mph; it could only make things worse. What the food companies needed was a set of standards for salt, with different levels allowed for different types of foods. And those standards had to cover thousands of food items on grocery shelves.

Angell discovered that another government had created standards like that. The equivalent of the FDA in the United Kingdom, the Food Standards Agency, working with food companies, had divided the most important food items into eighty-five categories. They measured the amount of salt in each category, set salt-reduction targets in each category, and then asked the food companies to commit to meeting those targets gradually over time. The big food companies had made real changes:

Heinz cut sodium by 19 percent in all its canned products, Kellogg's cut the sodium in cornflakes by 25 percent, and Kraft cut the sodium in cheese spreads and snacks by a third. Only a few years into the program, people in the U.K. were taking in 9 percent less sodium without even noticing it.

During 2007 and 2008 Silver and Angell quietly invited representatives from a few major food manufacturers to chat about sodium. Lowering sodium levels in food wouldn't be easy, the representatives said, but it was possible. They made a key request, though. Big manufacturers didn't make different versions of food for different cities. They made food. Any changes they might make would have to be national. The federal government, not New York City, should do the asking. The food companies probably figured that, since the federal government would do nothing, that request would make the issue go away.

. . .

On a gray day in late October 2008, Tom Frieden, Christina Chang, Mary Bassett, Lynn Silver, Sonia Angell, and Frieden's assistant Kelly Christ sat at round, linen-covered tables in the blue ballroom of Gracie Mansion for a lunch of grilled salmon, green salad, and unsweetened tea. Joining them were thirty-four representatives of seventeen of America's major food companies and their trade associations. They had come to hear what the mayor of New York had to say about salt.

The health department staff had struggled for months to hold this gathering. After some forty years of inaction on salt, they didn't want just another conversation. Frieden had labored over every word of the invitation. He wanted the tone to be a little ambiguous: a friendly invitation over an unstated threat. "I know that [company name] is committed to making its products healthier," it said. "I hope to discuss with you and other food industry leaders setting and implementing voluntary standards to reduce salt content." I imagined the CEOs puzzling over that. How could "standards" be voluntary?

Frieden wanted to talk directly with decision makers. He sent the companies' CEOs an e-mail after the invitation, saying that the initiative would succeed only "if there is commitment at the highest levels. For this reason I urge you to personally attend the meeting. If you are unable to join Mayor Bloomberg, please send a representative who is authorized to make commitments on your company's behalf."

The tone came through. One executive, speaking later anonymously to the *Times*, said, "I would say the invitations to come to Gracie Mansion weren't very inviting. . . . There was definitely a feeling of 'Don't make us shame you.'" An industry insider we spoke to saw "high levels of suspicion and concern that companies are heading into a trap."

In a later interview with the *Times*, Frieden was more direct. "If there's not progress in a few years, we'll have to consider other options, like legislation." Even with federal preemption, could New York City somehow *require* companies to limit the sodium in food sold within its boundaries? No one at the health department knew for sure. But then neither did the food industry, and the health department team wanted to make the most of that uncertainty.

Mayor Bloomberg was the attraction at the meeting. The city health department lacked the clout of the FDA, but it had on its side the nation's biggest voice in health. Showcasing Bloomberg for this particular initiative carried a risk, though—he *loved* salt. "He salts his *bacon*," Frieden told me. When the newspapers got wind of this initiative, they would be unable to resist writing about the billionaire who loved salt for himself but forced bad-tasting food on everyone else. Bloomberg especially loved to snack on Cheez-Its crackers. They were the perfectly balanced snack food, he told Frieden, with enough fat to clog your arteries and then enough salt to push the blood through.

Sonia Angell had figured out how to deal with the problem of Bloomberg's taste for salt. Most sodium is dissolved within food, but most of the taste zing happens when your tongue hits salt on a food's surface. In one study, researchers put a group of eleven students in a research lab for thirteen weeks and, without telling them, varied the amount of salt cooked in their food. During the entire study, the students had saltshakers at the table. When the researchers cut the salt content in the food by half, the students compensated by sprinkling more salt from the shakers, but only enough to replace a fraction of what the researchers had removed. Net, the students ate 30 percent less sodium and were just as satisfied. The sodium the health department would be asking companies to remove from food was often the sodium people didn't taste. And if people, like Bloomberg, wanted to use a saltshaker, they could sprinkle away and still come out ahead.

For the Gracie Mansion meeting, Bloomberg's speechwriters had figured that the best way to manage the problem was to spotlight it. "Let me start with a confession," Bloomberg's script said. "I love salty foods—really love them. I never eat fries or popcorn without a liberal sprinkling of salt. Despite all of the evidence linking salt to high blood pressure, my health commissioner actually condones this behavior! That's because the real salt in our diets—some eighty percent of it—comes from prepared foods."

But that afternoon, Bloomberg did what he usually did—he said whatever came into his head. Cheez-Its, he told the nation's food industry. That's what he really loved. If he could, he'd mash up Cheez-Its, put them in a saltshaker, and sprinkle them over his pizza. The Cheez-Its manufacturer applauded.

Frieden laid out the health department's plan to the companies. Their goal was to cut sodium levels in the entire food supply by 25 percent in five years. They would meet that goal by setting targets for sodium levels in the most important food categories and then ask the companies to commit to meet them. The targets would be "substantive, achievable, gradual, voluntary, and measurable." Representatives from the World Health Organization then summarized actions on salt that were under way in several European countries, and a woman from the U.K.'s Food Standards Agency showed how they had succeeded.

In response, "the industry was very polite," said Silver. The representatives admitted that sodium was a problem. But they warned that their customers would reject any food that tasted bad or even tasted just different. "They said they were looking at it, studying ways to do it, but wanted to do it themselves."

The health department team didn't want individual companies to work on the problem on their own. That's what had failed for so many years. The team wanted commitments and open measurement. Frieden asked the executives to send a follow-up letter in which they would "commit to participating in an iterative process by which targets will be created, goals will be set, and progress will be measured."

Afterward the health department team was ebullient. They didn't have any commitments in hand, but they had pulled off a crucial first step. The nation's food giants had shown up to a meeting called by a city health department; they were agreeing on the fundamental problem and what needed to be done about it. "People really took seriously that we were in the mayor's mansion and that the mayor cared about this," one staffer said later. Mary Bassett e-mailed me that the meeting had been "pitch perfect. . . . Tom was brilliant as a facilitator [and] the mayor charmingly off message." And the threat had been heard, Bassett wrote, with just enough "subtle reminders of regulatory potential."

Afterward Christina Chang and others from the health department went out to a bar to celebrate. With margaritas in glasses rimmed with salt.

. . .

The food companies may have had other reasons for listening to Bloomberg and Frieden. Even though the mayor was nearing the end his second term, it looked like neither he nor his health commissioner was going away.

Earlier that year Bloomberg had finally shut the door on a presidential run. His top political adviser Kevin Sheekey had been agitating for it for years. Bloomberg had the ability to do it his own way, entirely with his own money, like Ross Perot only smarter. Bloomberg had abandoned the Republican Party so he could run as an independent if he wanted to. Sheekey and his staff had researched what it would take to get on the ballot in all fifty states; they had sounded out potential supporters and run polls, while Bloomberg traveled around the country expressing candidatelike opinions on the state of the nation. But in the end, the mayor was too realistic to jump. He told colleagues that a Jewish, pro-choice, progay-marriage, pro-gun-control New Yorker polled at about 10 percent.

Soon afterward, though, Bloomberg's staff polled New Yorkers about his seeking a third term as mayor. That would require the City Council to pass a law revising the city's term limits, which the voters had approved. The polls said that while Bloomberg was very popular, New Yorkers strongly opposed him changing that law. Ignoring his advisers, who pleaded with him not to do it, Bloomberg lobbied the City Council to rewrite the law. The Salt Summit occurred less than a week after that vote, which had cleared the way for him to run for a third term. Bloomberg likely would be mayor of New York City for another four years.

The Salt Summit also happened days before the 2008 presidential election, as Democratic candidate Barack Obama was holding a good lead in the polls. Rumors were circulating that an Obama administration might appoint Frieden as director of the CDC or some other prominent federal health job. A smart food company CEO would recognize that it was a good idea to hear what Frieden had to say.

Frieden must have had a federal position on his mind. One day in early 2008, when I was working as his adviser, he had asked me if I wanted to spend a day shadowing him. I turned him down. I was busy, and happily so, working with Mary Bassett and her staff on problems like obesity and high salt levels in food. I liked working behind the scenes while Frieden fought the political battles. Then after I finished my year there, he asked if I could continue to help him part time, and I agreed. We talked on the phone regularly, and I made occasional trips to the city. During one of them, he asked me if I might be interested in becoming the next New York City health commissioner.

His question caught me off guard. I had wanted to direct a city health department, but it had never occurred to me that I might get the chance to run the most prominent one in the nation. I told Frieden that I was excited at the opportunity to make a difference in people's lives, but I was also scared that I'd screw it up. Making decisions about public health worried me less than being able to do the political maneuvering to make the decisions stick. "I'm an excellent epidemiologist, a so-so manager, and a lousy politician," I told him. And I put him off.

. . .

After the Salt Summit, Frieden got many letters from the food companies, but they didn't say what he wanted to hear. Nearly all of them wrote that they were already working on salt reduction. One even wrote, "Last December we announced that our sodium reduction efforts have successfully removed nearly three million pounds of salt from American diets annually." Claims like that, though, were exactly the problem. There was no way to verify them, and despite the impressive numbers, Americans' intake of sodium appeared to be increasing. The companies' pledges were frustratingly evasive; one executive wrote that his company was "committed to helping consumers achieve a healthy lifestyle and we look forward to working with you to achieve this goal."

And with only a few exceptions, the food companies circled their wagons and redirected Frieden to their trade group, the Grocery Manufacturers Association (GMA). The GMA was doing what trade associations are paid to do with proposed government actions: pretend to help while working to neutralize them. Before and after the Gracie Mansion meeting, GMA vice president Bob Earl was on the phone almost daily with health department staff. He questioned the purpose, insisted that the food company CEOs should not attend, and demanded in advance an agenda, a list of invitees, and a list of those agreeing to come. He asked that the health department expand the meetings to include grocery stores, restaurants, delis, and institutional food vendors. He said the process "must also consider other policy issues and initiatives related to labeling, consumer education, and research funding on taste and salt replacements." Less than a month after the Salt Summit, he announced that his association would hold its own conference to develop its own salt-reduction plan. And at every step, he demanded that the process be slowed down.

The health department was also stirring up another industry. The Salt Institute is an association of companies that sell salt, like Morton and Cargill. ("There's a lobby for *everything*," a congressional staffer once told me.) The "institute" devotes most of its effort to showing that reducing the amount of salt in foods would be dangerous. David McCarron, an adjunct professor at the University of California at Davis who is paid by the Salt Institute, visited the health department in January 2009 to present his argument. Sodium has a "minimal" effect on blood pressure, he said. People have a sodium "set point," so that if you cut the amount of sodium in their food, they will just eat more food to compensate and become obese. On the other hand, people who already have severe heart disease can die if you abruptly cut back their sodium intake. He said the issue needed more research, in particular a massive, years-long study in which people are assigned to high- and low-salt diets and the researchers measure which group survives longer.

Lynn Silver called the whole argument "specious." A study of the kind the Salt Institute proposed would be impractical (who would stick to their diets?) and—many experts would say—unethical, so it would never be done. That, I figured, was why the Salt Institute called for it. The claims of the salt doubters reminded me of decades-long arguments that some prominent, industry-funded scientists made about lead in paint and gasoline. The risks aren't clear, they said; the studies are flawed. Meanwhile, hundreds of thousands of children were getting brain damage from lead poisoning.

Silver and her team ignored McCarron. But despite the obvious corporate interest behind the Salt Institute's argument, they had reason to worry. The argument had just enough ring of science to provide cover for food companies that didn't want to budge.

. . .

Six months after the Salt Summit, Frieden, Silver, Angell and rest of the salt team met at the health department's headquarters with eight food company representatives. They had come to talk about ketchup. The team had started with ketchup because it looked like the simplest food category, and they needed simplicity because the whole exercise was proving to be very complicated.

The salt team had two tasks: group food items into categories and then choose a sodium target in each category. The United Kingdom had done that, and the salt team hoped to make minor adjustments to the U.K.'s categories and targets. They would group foods that were similar (like sandwich bread and English muffins) but separate foods that were different enough in taste or recipe to have sharply different sodium levels (like doughnuts at 300 mg versus waffles at 570 mg per 100 grams). The salt team didn't care about specific foods as much as the total sodium sold in a food category. An extremely salty gourmet cracker with a niche market was less dangerous than a moderately salty generic cracker eaten by half the country.

The team's measure of progress, then, took into account both the sodium levels in each food item and the amount of sales. Having the metric be a "sales-weighted average" would give the food companies many ways to meet a reduction target; they could phase out a high-salt product, introduce a new low-salt product, or cut the salt in continuing products. But it made the calculations complicated and dependent on data on both sodium levels and sales.

Angell gave Christine Curtis the job of building the database to measure that progress. Curtis, a tall, sandy-haired woman, had come to city government as a policy intern a few years earlier. She had a head for numbers and was unflappable, and she soon became the agency's salt expert. The commercial food database that she built was more complete than any in the nation, and her calculations of sodium levels in food categories were the first that anyone—especially the food companies—had ever seen.

Silver and Angell's plan was to meet with the dominant manufacturers for each food category to discuss proposed targets, then choose final targets and ask the companies to pledge to meet them. Ketchup seemed like a good starting place because its sodium level was different enough from that of other condiments that Curtis thought it should be in a category all by itself.

A 14-ounce bottle of a leading brand of ketchup contained a little over 1½ teaspoons of salt. A single tablespoon of ketchup that you might put on a hamburger delivered about 10 percent of your sodium budget for an entire day. Curtis now proposed to the ketchup manufacturers targets that would cut the salt in ketchup by one-tenth in 2011 and one-quarter in 2013. Both those proposals were less stringent than the targets already set for ketchup by the U.K.

After Curtis finished presenting the proposal, the meeting erupted. Bob Earl from GMA wanted to see the entire list of proposed categories, the schedule of meetings, and a description of the steps to create the final targets. A major ketchup manufacturer demanded to know why the health department was picking on ketchup first when ketchup was such a small contributor to sodium intake. Other ketchup manufacturers wanted ketchup grouped with barbecue sauce and salsa. Then they argued that salt in ketchup wasn't just about taste. It also was a preservative, keeping food safe, and it kept the food stable on the shelf. Did the health department have any technical data on the impact lowering sodium levels in ketchup would have on safety? Representatives of one major manufacturer were "beside themselves," according to Chang, so much so that a man from a restaurant chain turned to them and said, "Guys, in the end, it's just ketchup."

And that was the simplest category. The next, crackers, was much more complicated. Saltines, peanut-butter-filled crackers, flavored snack crackers (like Bloomberg's Cheez-Its) were in; graham crackers, Melba toast, and hard bread sticks were out. Just five saltine crackers delivered 6 to 9 percent of a daily sodium budget. At the cracker meeting, Curtis proposed cutting the average sodium level by 15 percent by 2011 and another 15 percent by 2013. Both targets would be less stringent than the U.K. targets, and many popular crackers sold in the United States already met them.

The cracker makers raised their own complaints. Snack, butter, and filled crackers couldn't be lumped together. Sodium was used in crackers not just in the form of salt but also in as baking soda for leavening. Healthier crackers that used whole wheat needed more leavening, which meant more sodium. Salt also was used in crackers for texture, and companies had to alter the amount of salt in a recipe according to how much gluten was in the wheat flour, which changed according to when the wheat had been harvested. The salt sprinkled on top of crackers often fell off and settled to the bottom of the box, so the companies shouldn't be blamed for it. And they were competing with "private label" manufacturers who weren't in the conversation.

Between March and July 2009, Silver, Angell, and Curtis held meetings on thirty-two different food categories, squabbling with food companies over breakfast cereal, frozen snacks, potato chips, popcorn, bread and rolls, canned tuna, entrée sauces, soft cheese, hard cheese, canned beans, soups, salad dressing, and salted butter. Making arguments about taste, leavening, and texture, the companies griped that the targets were too aggressive. Even though they had said for decades that they were working on cutting salt levels, the companies complained that New York City was unrealistic in asking them to make changes over two or four years.

The packaged food companies also insisted that they were competing with restaurants. So in January 2009, Frieden and his team held a second Salt Summit for restaurants. Thirteen chains showed up. The restaurant summit spun off its own fractious meetings for categories like hamburgers, cheeseburgers, burritos, cheese pizza, soups, and breaded seafood. Most restaurants hadn't even begun to think about lowering salt levels. Even beyond the technical problems, "the restaurants were tough," said Silver. "They were already pissed off at us about calorie labeling."

None of this was going to be easy.

. . .

In the spring of 2009, after Barack Obama nominated Kathleen Sebelius for secretary of health and human services, Frieden heard that he would be offered the job of director of the CDC. He asked me again if I would replace him in New York City. This time I said yes.

Four days later a public health crisis erupted. The government in Mexico announced it was shutting schools and other public places in Mexico City to stop the spread of what it called a new swine flu virus, which had already killed sixty-one people. On the same day, the New York City health department heard that some seventy-five high school students from Queens who had just returned from a spring break in Cancún were sick with fever. Within two days, the WHO declared a public health emergency over a new strain of influenza virus. If the nearly 10 percent death rate among victims from initial Mexican reports were to hold up, this could be the deadly pandemic that public health experts had been dreading for decades. It would be the job of New York City's health commissioner to protect the city from the infection. That meant Frieden had to decide whether to quarantine people who were sick, and what advice to give New Yorkers about getting vaccinated, taking antiviral drugs, and the risks of using the subway. Because the city was the first U.S. location hit by the virus, the rest of the nation was watching.

For a week Frieden was the center of a national media frenzy. Then I flew to New York to interview in Gracie Mansion with Mayor Bloomberg and Deputy Mayors Patti Harris and Linda Gibbs. By the time HHS was ready to announce Frieden as CDC director and Bloomberg was ready to name me health commissioner, the H1N1 influenza epidemic had spread from New York to much of the United States and many other countries. The disease seemed to be hitting children especially hard, and Frieden had begun closing schools. While most infected people were recovering, one assistant principal was near death. Suddenly, it mattered to many people who was in charge of health in New York City.

On Monday, May 18, feeling a little like a man headed to the firing squad, I followed Bloomberg and Gibbs to stand behind the podium in City Hall's Blue Room. The room, named for its cobalt carpeting, walls, and drapes, was outfitted with an ornate chandelier in the center, a platform for video cameras in the back, and a large portrait of Alexander Hamilton at the front. "Tom assumes this vital post at a time when public health is obviously on the front burner," said the mayor. I looked up from the podium and saw a sea of reporters' faces and a battery of TV news cameras. I read a few words I had written down. "My goal as the New York City health commissioner," I said, "will be to continue to make advances against the leading causes of death for New Yorkers today, such as smoking and obesity."

"The speed with which a replacement was chosen underscores the importance of the post, as well as the urgency of the H1N1 flu outbreak that Dr. Farley must confront," wrote the *Times*, which—thank goodness—called me "an infectious disease specialist." I had never been so nervous in my life.

PART TWO

10

"All I could think of was,
welcome to New York."

On Monday morning, June 8, 2009, I walked into the corner
office at the health department and sat behind what I still
thought of as Tom Frieden's desk. I felt as if I were taking over as manager of the Yankees after they had won the World Series seven years in a
row. Even if I won big, it would look like inertia. Still, this would be my
chance, an opportunity not only to save lives but also to change the way
people fought disease.

That first day I invited a dozen deputies in for a little speech. Like
Frieden, I told them, I loved numbers and would be driven by data and
scientific evidence. I wanted to go after unhealthy behaviors by addressing the conditions that fostered them. Often that would mean writing
new rules, rules that would need approval by the Board of Health, the
City Council, or other policy-making bodies. Although Frieden and I
had gone through similar training and often thought alike, our personali-
ties were very different. Frieden plays squash, a sport that is frenetic and
competitive. I'm a long-distance runner: steady and contemplative. I tried
to give my team a sense of how I would be different. I wouldn't micro-
manage. In an agency that covered this much territory, I simply couldn't.
I preferred to spend chunks of time in the early days with each deputy, so
that they and I would understand each other's strategy—and then get out

of the way. I wouldn't yell, but they shouldn't mistake my quiet manner for lack of determination.

I was open about my weaknesses. My management experience in government was limited to a few years running programs in Louisiana's health department. I hadn't been chosen for my management skills, I said. Without their help in managing this huge department and navigating the turbulent political seas of City Hall, I told the deputies, I would fail, and so would they.

Later Christina Chang, who initially stayed on as my chief of staff, gave me her first piece of advice: Don't talk like that. The health department was hierarchical. The staff were accustomed to a leader who was "kind of arrogant"; I would only undercut myself by showing weakness. It was like that in City Hall, too. There, Frieden "was seen sometimes as stubborn and obstinate and kind of a bully," she said, but that protected the health department. In the mayor's office, "if you admit weakness in anything, you will get ridden roughshod."

I considered the obstacles and the opportunities in front of me. I faced a problem in common with every city health director: I would be pressed by the public's expectations and fears, which would make it difficult to push the actions that save the most lives.

Most city health departments, most of the time, are nearly invisible to the public. They quietly do things that residents take for granted, like inspecting restaurants, catching stray dogs, treating people with tuberculosis, and keeping the drinking water safe. As hidden as the traditional health department programs are, they touch on raw nerves. On any day, any program can explode in the public eye, such as when a popular restaurant is overrun by rats, a well-heeled group catches salmonella, or a kindergarten teacher is diagnosed with drug-resistant tuberculosis. When problems like these erupt, the ensuing outrage can damage the department, the health director, and the mayor.

In my first few months on the job, the H1N1 influenza pandemic seemed poised to roil the city and ruin me. The nation's public health agencies had long expected a new killer strain of the flu virus to jump from pigs or birds to humans. Health departments had developed their response plans: until a vaccine arrived, doctors would treat the sick with antiviral medications—drugs that were only partially effective—and health directors would try to slow the spread by separating sick people from healthy people. Even if everyone executed those plans well, however, the infection could easily sweep the world and kill tens of millions. The people hit the hardest would be the elderly.

But the new H1N1 influenza strain refused to follow the script. The infection raced through the nation, but it mainly struck children and young adults, most of whom recovered quickly. (Older people escaped probably because they were immune after infection from similar strains many influenza seasons earlier.) Few if anyone in public health had envisioned an influenza pandemic that infected legions of young people but killed very few. We realized only gradually that we had escaped the Big One, but then we didn't have a useful playbook. We were caught between underreacting and overreacting.

Tom Frieden and I struggled with whether to close schools, which studies suggested could slow an influenza epidemic, buying time while a vaccine was being developed. Shortly before I started, the ill assistant principal had died of the new flu, followed soon afterward by a child in an elementary school. Many parents and teachers panicked and pressed to close the schools. But other parents, seeing most children recover after two days of mild fever, pressed just as hard to keep the schools open; they had to go to work, and sending their children to a babysitter's home packed with other children hardly seemed safer. At first Frieden had closed a few schools where many children were becoming sick. But as it became clearer that this epidemic of influenza was not particularly deadly, he and then I left the schools open. The new virus retreated in the summer of 2010.

It returned the following winter, but by that time we had a vaccine. The health department shipped the vaccine to doctors throughout the city and set up special vaccine clinics. Initially some people desperately wanted a vaccine that they were unable to get; after dealing with that, we quickly ran into the opposite problem: most people feared a new vaccine more than a now-familiar virus. In the end, the nation discarded millions of unwanted doses of vaccine, and the new H1N1 influenza virus merged into the annual influenza ebb and flow. The much-feared pandemic killed far fewer New Yorkers than influenza did in a typical year. And the New York City health department got through the bizarre episode with its reputation intact.

· · ·

All city health directors handle crises like this, and they all manage long-standing programs to try to avoid them. For many city health directors, that is their entire job. But for me, to *only* maintain those programs and stamp out flare-ups would be to fail. Today the long-standing health programs have very little to do with how healthy we are. Nothing about killing rats or closing a deli serving contaminated potato salad prevents people from catching heart disease, cancer, or diabetes.

Frieden had dealt with that contradiction by redefining the job of the city health director. To him, the job was not about *providing services*. It was about *preventing needless deaths*. If people were dying from heart attacks or cancer or diabetes, then that's where the health department should be.

Prevention is always a tough sell. When people get sick, they demand to be cared for. They want a doctor to write a prescription and tell them it will be all right, and they want a nurse to ease their discomforts. On the other hand, people think only rarely about prevention; when they do, they usually view it as a matter of personal responsibility, not something to demand of others. Health directors in other cities wanted to redirect their agencies to prevent chronic diseases as much Frieden did, but they were straitjacketed by tight budgets, timid mayors, and the curse of expectations. But Frieden had had backing from Mayor Bloomberg to make that radical turn.

His health department couldn't prevent chronic diseases by itself, though. It had the legal authority to close restaurants and quarantine people, but it had no such weapons to fight smoking, unhealthy eating, or physical inactivity. Reducing those risks had required Frieden to tell New Yorkers what to do. He had pressed bills on City Council members, published instructions for doctors, and posted commands in subway ads for every other New Yorker. Creating those directives required the department to gather and analyze data, write reports, craft recommendations, draft bills, and produce ads, and then use all channels of modern communication to circulate the products. So over the course of seven and a half years, Frieden had transformed the health department, establishing thriving units to do epidemiology, chronic disease prevention, legal analysis, and communications.

For years before I arrived, I had been arguing that chronic diseases are preventable by making healthier choices easier. It's a simple idea that is difficult to realize. Powerful forces resist the changes that prevent today's killer diseases. Too often the architects of our day-to-day world are companies marketing unhealthy products, like cigarettes, junk food, and junk beverages. If I wanted to make healthy choices easier, I had to change government rules to protect people from that marketing. And changing the rules inevitably provokes the companies doing the marketing into battle. People in public health have to pick their battles, to find chinks in the armor of strong opponents. Nonetheless, watching Frieden had made it clear to me that saving lives requires fighting.

That makes prevention even tougher to sell to politicians. Championing prevention means taking on political skirmishes that mayors or governors may lose, while few constituents cheer them on. Even if the initiatives succeed in preventing needless deaths, and even if the citizens are grateful for what didn't happen, the payoff comes well beyond the next election. Politically, public health is more trouble than it's worth. Because of that, public health officials are usually shut out of power. We attend conferences where we blather on about what *should* happen but almost never get opportunities to determine what *will* happen.

Now I had such an opportunity, but I knew it wouldn't last long. The mayor's support, his sway with the City Council, and the authority of the Board of Health were a fleeting alignment of stars. I owed it to public health not to squander it.

The stakes were higher even than the lives of eight million New Yorkers. New York is a global megacity and a media hub. Local stories can quickly catapult to become national or international events. When those stories are controversial, people everywhere else notice. By 2009 people around the country and around the world were paying attention to the New York City health department. Before New York City passed its smoke-free air law, only California and a few health-conscious towns in Colorado and Massachusetts had had smoke-free bars. After New York City—and then its suburban counties, and then the state—went smoke-free, similar laws spread across the country. By 2007 cities like Houston, Texas, and Columbus, Ohio, had smoke-free restaurants and bars. By early 2010 smoke-free-air laws were in place in thirty-two states, including the nation's tobacco capital, North Carolina. The trend was also sweeping Europe. In 2002, after the Irish delegation interrogated Christina Chang about how the New York team had passed its law, groups from other European countries followed, in person or on the phone. Norway and the Netherlands passed comprehensive smoke-free-air laws shortly after Ireland did. Sweden, Italy, and Spain followed. By 2007 Britain and even cigarette-loving France had smoke-free bars.

New York City's trans fat ban also traveled quickly. As soon as the story hit the press, other cities began calling the health department for help on how to write similar regulations. Within three months of our Board of Health vote, the Philadelphia City Council voted to restrict trans fats. Seattle passed a restaurant ban a few months later; it was followed later that year by suburban counties near New York and Baltimore, and by the entire state of California in 2008. And by the end of 2008, McDonald's, Burger King, Subway, Starbucks, and several other big chains had announced that they would stop using trans fats in all their restaurants nationwide.

Just a few days after I started the job, Lynn Silver e-mailed me with news about restaurant calorie counts. Senator Tom Harkin (D-Iowa) wanted to wrap his bill on mandatory calorie labeling in chain restaurants into President Obama's health care reform bill. Harkin's staff had called Silver to make sure the bill wouldn't interfere with our calorie-labeling rule. After checking, she told them there was no major conflict, and restaurant menu labeling ended up in the Affordable Care Act. The calorie counts will one day go nationwide, too.

. . .

Often new department heads replace the people who report to them. I didn't have a choice. Within a few weeks of my starting, two deputy commissioners told me they were leaving—they felt burned out, they said, and needed a change—and the chief operating officer followed Tom Frieden to CDC. Even before I arrived, and shortly before Frieden told people that he was leaving, Mary Bassett had quit. "Tom is an enormously dedicated person," she had told me. "He works heart and soul to accomplish goals. And he gets very involved. His involvement always adds value to everything that we do. . . . But the downside is also that." Her frustration that Frieden made all the decisions ate at her. Years later she was more direct: "I hated working for Tom."

To fill in her position running the Division of Health Promotion and Disease Prevention, I promoted Andy Goodman, a mild-mannered pediatrician who had been with the health department for twenty-five years and was then directing the Harlem office. Goodman was another liberal who had traveled to Nicaragua after the 1980s revolution and had even helped Frieden edit his Central America health newsletter. Bassett's division oversaw the fifteen-hundred-staff Office of School Health; its chief had to have diplomacy in dealing with those staff and with the city's enormous Department of Education, a diplomacy that I thought Goodman had. Lynn Silver had applied for the position too and felt insulted that I gave it to Goodman. They clashed, and the change set up trouble for me later.

. . .

Several New York City news outlets wanted to interview the new guy. Geoff Cowley, a science writer for *Newsweek* whom Frieden had hired as the agency's communications director, and who was himself still learning how to deal with the scrappy City Hall press corps, advised me to do the interviews. They would give me a chance to frame my agenda and might buy me some goodwill with reporters, which I'd need for the battles ahead.

Only gradually did I come to understand the weird symbiotic relationship between news outlets and elected officials, which others seemed to grasp intuitively. It's not just vanity that compels mayors, governors, and presidents to go to great lengths to look like winners on the evening news. Those elected officials ultimately draw their power from voters, who know their leaders almost entirely by how the press portrays them. Mayors need good coverage. Every day news outlets have the option of showing a mayor solving problems, fighting evil, and caring for people like you and me—or acting petty, defeated, or overbearing. Those news outlets, especially during the Internet era, are fighting for as many readers' and viewers' eyeballs as they can get. They need stories every day— the juicier the better.

Unfortunately, juicy stories usually make mayors look bad. The conflicting needs of the press and the mayor led to a daily wrestling match between reporters and the City Hall press office. As Geoff Cowley put it, the press team was always "jockeying to get the kind of coverage you want from people who are basically out to screw you."

At the health department, we couldn't avoid getting dragged into this wrestling match. We put out reports on the health problems of New Yorkers that told people and organizations what they should do to avoid them; we believed publishing those reports was a key part of our job. We also proposed ideas to Bloomberg that had built-in opponents. The City Hall press office seemed to groan whenever my staff showed up. Why were we yakking about diabetes or arthritis—problems that Mayor Bloomberg couldn't fix? Why were we picking fights that the mayor might lose? They tended to consider us as troublemakers. In turn, we considered the press office meddlesome. We understood that the mayor had to spend his political capital wisely, but what better way to spend political capital than to save lives? Or as Lyndon Johnson said when his aides warned him that the civil rights bill would be too controversial, "What the hell's the presidency for?"

Every day the newspapers set the tone for how the press in general would cover an issue. The television and radio stations usually followed along. That made the City Hall press team particularly obsessed with how the newspapers framed a story. Of the major daily papers, *The New York Times* and *The Wall Street Journal* saw themselves mainly as highbrow national papers that dipped into some local stories. There were two local tabloids, the arch-conservative *New York Post* (a Rupert Murdoch production) and the left-leaning *Daily News*.

Other than glimpsing headlines like "HEADLESS BODY IN TOPLESS BAR" as I walked by newsstands, I had never read the tabloids, so in the first couple of days I scanned them to learn what they were about. On my first day on the job, the *Post* informed New Yorkers about a man who had maintained an active membership for a decade in a women-only gym, an ex-con who was suing a prison nurse who had ignored his painful fifty-five-hour erection, and a special rescue team that had rappelled down a cliff in Connecticut to rescue what had turned out to be a mannequin. It was like reading the funny pages, only not as funny.

I was wary of the interviews, so in advance I wrote out talking points and answers to tough questions. Geoff Cowley told me that the press was frustrated that Frieden had been fiercely protective of his private life, so if I could open up about myself, even just a little, I would win some badly needed goodwill.

My first interview was with Adam Lisberg, a reporter for the *Daily News*. We talked about my approach to public health for about fifteen minutes, during which I was proud of how closely I kept to my script. My goal, I told Lisberg, was to prevent the leading causes of death in New York City by making the city a healthier place in which to live. The indoor smoking ban, the tough TV antismoking ads, and the trans fat ban had been part of that effort, and New Yorkers were benefiting from them. "I don't think anybody feels a great loss in not having trans fat in their foods," I said.

Toward the end, Lisberg said he understood that I liked to exercise and even had ridden my bike to work in New Orleans. Yes, I told him, I liked to run and ride a bike. Would I be biking to work in New York City? he asked.

Sure, I said.

Even in Manhattan?

"At the moment in Manhattan, no," I said, because I was a little uncomfortable with the safety in traffic.

He smiled faintly and left.

Gotcha. The story ran the next day under the massive headline "NEW YORK HEALTH BOSS SCARED TO CYCLE ON OUR STREETS." "The man in charge of making New Yorkers healthier says riding your bike is a great way to do it—but he's not sure he's ready to try it on city streets," it opened. I'm sure it infuriated Janette Sadik-Khan, the transportation commissioner who was enduring her own hazing by the tabloids for painting bike lanes on city streets. She was restrained, though, telling the *Daily News*, "I certainly look forward to riding around the streets of New York with the new health commissioner."

I thought the story was silly, but the press office took it dead seriously. And sure enough, for the next three months, in nearly every interview I did, even if it was about the influenza pandemic, at some point the reporter would get around to asking me a variation of "So, Commissioner, are you finally ready to ride your bike in New York?" The only way I could kill the story was to ride my bike to work in Manhattan, bringing a *Daily News* reporter along with me.

The day the story first appeared, the *Daily News* even pressed Bloomberg about it. The mayor said, "When I saw it in the paper . . . all I could think of was, welcome to New York."

11

"They can't even be
bothered to sue us?"

When I started at the health department, the tobacco team was waiting eagerly for me. They had an idea ready to launch.

New York City was already doing everything that most smoking prevention experts around the country were calling for: high cigarette taxes, a smoke-free air law, a Smokers' Quitline, and tough television ads. Nonetheless one in six adults in New York City still smoked, and the agency still counted smoking as the city's biggest killer. We needed to do more, but we no longer had a trail to follow.

At Tom Frieden's prodding, the tobacco team had spawned many ideas. Sarah Perl, who now ran tobacco control, considered expanding the Smoke-Free Air Act. It now banned smoking in public places indoors, but people still smoked in crowded places outdoors, giving others a small but daily dose of hazardous secondhand smoke and—more important—broadcasting that smoking was normal and even cool. Perl considered smoke-free train platforms, bus shelters, college dormitories, college campuses, parks, beaches, and building entrances.

Perl and her staff also believed that smoking rates would fall faster if the city had fewer stores selling cigarettes. Eleven thousand grocery stores, pharmacies, and bodegas with tobacco licenses packed the city, with many neighborhoods having several in a single block. Perl considered asking the City Council to cut the number of licenses by half. Or to restrict cigarette sales to stores that sold tobacco only, just as New York State restricts sales of wine and spirits to liquor stores. Frieden had devoured the ideas but hadn't taken them to City Hall because he wasn't convinced that the health payoffs were worth the political battles and legal risks.

In 2002 Donna Shelley had told him, "Keep your eye on the enemy. It's the tobacco industry." The problem the department faced was not tobacco itself but instead the *marketing* of smoking. Philip Morris, R.J. Reynolds, and Lorillard did everything they legally could to get more people to smoke more. It's what the executives were paid to do. Over the decades, as society tightened the rules on cigarettes, the tobacco companies had answered by rechanneling their marketing dollars. When I was in grade school in the 1960s, they ran relentless ads in newspapers, in magazines, on billboards, and on television. I can still sing the "Come up to the Kool taste!" jingle. From then through the early 2000s federal regulations and a state attorneys general lawsuit had eliminated television, billboard, and most print ads.

Nonetheless, from 1986 to 2011 the tobacco companies quadrupled the money they spent on advertising and promotion, to nearly $10 billion a year. The companies poured nearly 95 percent of that fortune into retail stores, buying point-of-sale ads, discount coupons, price reductions, buy-one-get-one-free promotions, and payoffs to stores for displaying packs in enticing ways or hitting sales targets. Those shiny packs, ads, and discount signs stood immediately behind the stores' cash registers in what public health people called "power walls," which attracted the eyes of children and lured smokers who were trying to quit to buy on impulse. All those grocery stores, pharmacies, and bodegas in New York City were now the hyperaggressive marketing arm of the tobacco industry. Tobacco executives were experts in how to sell smoking. If they were spending billions on discounts and power walls in retail stores, it must be worth it.

In 2009 Congress had passed a law giving the FDA the authority to regulate tobacco but it left to states and cities the power to regulate the "time, place, and manner" of cigarette sales. That opened a chink in the armor that health department lawyer Anne Pearson spotted. A cigarette pack in the United States carried a puny warning label, using text only, which smokers could see only after they bought the pack. Other countries were covering nearly half of the pack with ugly pictures showing diseased lungs or stained teeth. When the pictures appeared, smokers were more likely to notice the warnings and consider quitting.

Pearson's idea was to force the cigarette retailers to post pictures like that, not on the packs but on warning signs alongside the cigarette racks. There smokers would see the images before they bought cigarettes, and some might reconsider. The Board of Health could pass the rule, Pearson thought, so it wouldn't require rounding up votes from City Council members who were lobbied by Philip Morris and the convenience stores. Pearson had pitched the idea to Tom Frieden just before he left. "His face kind of lit up," she said later. And he asked, "Really, we could do this!?"

When I heard the idea in my first meeting with the tobacco team, I practically jumped out of my chair. To me, the idea was bigger than just warning signs; going into retail stores meant opening up a new front in the war against the nation's biggest killer.

The Board of Health, which as health commissioner I now chaired, met just a week later, on my third week on the job. The board immediately warmed to the idea, too. We hadn't yet decided what the pictures on the warning signs would look like, and I wanted to downplay the ugliness of the images in the press, but reporters caught Sarah Perl while I was still running the board meeting, and she held forth with just the opposite. "You're going to see the grim realities of what it means to smoke," she told them. "You're going to see what a blackened lung looks like. You're going to see what mouth cancer looks like. You're going to see what it looks like when you have throat cancer."

Early the next morning I was stepping out of the shower when my BlackBerry rang with a call from Linda Gibbs, furious. The tabloid coverage was awful. We were going to force everyone to see "grisly" pictures, as big as three feet by three feet, whenever they went to a bodega to buy a carton of milk? The *Post* editorialized, "So what's next? Mandatory autopsy attendance?" Later that day, I had another conversation with her, and Gibbs was in bright spirits. She had shown Mayor Bloomberg the *Daily News* story, and he had shrugged. That's just the health department doing its job, he'd said.

We learned later that the type of pictures mattered a lot. Sarah Perl sent her researcher Beth Kilgore to learn what kind of images would work in bodegas. They mocked up six warning signs, ranging from just words to pictures of bloody, cancerous growths, and held focus groups with people who bought cigarettes at bodegas and with young people. Kilgore quickly learned that any warning sign had to pass the "sandwich test." In every group someone would say, "When I'm going in and buying a sandwich, I don't want to see this." The "gross" images failed the test. The text-only signs were far too easy to ignore.

But three pictures that she labeled "clinical" hit the sweet spot. They were a chest X-ray showing a blotchy lung cancer, a brain scan diagramming damage from a stroke, and an extracted tooth with smoking-related decay. Each sign said "Quit Smoking Today" and included the city's 311 Smokers' Quitline. "It grabs your attention," a younger smoker said. "And it's not gross, so it doesn't make you turn away. It does make you want to read more."

We expected that the tobacco companies would hate the warning sign rule. What company wants stores telling customers at the cash register not to buy its product? And at first, it looked like we were dead right. When the proposed rule was posted for public comment, we got an ominous memo from Arnold & Porter, the law firm that had fought us over restaurant calorie labeling and that now represented Altria (Philip Morris). The FDA now had the power to require pictorial warnings on cigarette packs, they wrote, so New York City should "refrain in the interim from issuing graphic health warning requirements on its own." The threat was that the federal law would preempt our local rule. And the Board of Health "would be exceeding its administrative authority by regulating in areas reserved for legislative policy judgment."

Altria was joined in criticizing the rule by the Food Industry Alliance (a trade group of grocery stores), the NYC Newsstand Operators Association, and the New York Association of Convenience Stores. The groups took offense that we wanted to warn people about the deadly drug they were selling. The signs would be too big, they wrote. The grocery stores argued that displaying the signs "is distasteful and runs counter to the positive shopping experience that a retailer seeks to create." The convenience stores followed: "If ghoulish pictures of black lungs dominate the view of our counter, they will be seen not only by adult tobacco smokers, but by non-smokers entering the store to buy milk, produce, candy, beverages, newspapers, lottery, and everything else we sell."

None of this surprised us, but it did serve notice for a battle. We shrank the warning signs to 12 by 12 inches at cash registers and 24 by 24 inches at tobacco displays but otherwise left the rule intact, and the Board of Health approved it. We started mailing out the "clinical" signs to tobacco sellers in the fall of 2009 and promised that the city would start enforcing the rule in January 2010.

Shortly before Christmas, Anne Pearson walked into a bodega and was excited to finally see the pictures posted at the counter. With so many cigarette sellers in the city, she realized that "the city was plastered with these really powerful images." But strangely, she was also embarrassed. It had been months since the rule passed, and the tobacco companies still hadn't filed a lawsuit. "I remember thinking, 'Oh my god, is this so unimportant, so ineffective that they can't even be bothered to sue us?'"

. . .

On November 3, 2009, Michael Bloomberg was elected mayor of New York City for the third time. He won by 51 to 46 percent over city comptroller Bill Thompson, who hadn't campaigned very hard. I was struck by the difference between Bloomberg's 63 percent approval rating and his 51 percent vote count. New Yorkers liked how he was running the city, but voters were angry that he had changed the law to run for a third term. He had four more years, but they might be rougher than the first eight.

I naïvely thought that, with no more elections in Bloomberg's future, his aides would be less resistant to ideas that were good for New Yorkers but bad in the press. In the summer of 2010, still thinking about the retail stores, I tried out two of the ideas that the tobacco team had worked on.

New York's City Hall is a graceful white structure, built in the early 1800s to serve as the center of government for the feverishly growing port city. It sits amid a small triangular park, a short walk from the health department. With steps leading to a portico in front, the building inside has two wings flanking a white marble rotunda. The mayor and his staff occupy one wing, and a large City Council chamber fills most of the other.

On the first floor of mayor's side is the Blue Room, used for decades for mayoral press conferences. On the second floor is a giant hearing room that Bloomberg had filled with cubicles and turned into his "Bull Pen"—a Wall Street trader–like office for him and his aides, with his desk dead center among them. Across the hall from the Bull Pen was the committee-of-the-whole room, known as the Cow, once capable of holding the entire City Council but now used for meetings with the mayor and his staff. The room contains a marble fireplace and is trimmed with green carpeting and gold drapes. In this room, next to a large, round mahogany table and under an ancient chandelier, I took Mayor Bloomberg through a slide presentation about cigarette marketing, pharmacies, and children.

San Francisco and Boston had just passed laws prohibiting the sale of cigarettes in pharmacies. Most independent pharmacies, managed by individual pharmacists, didn't sell cigarettes. But the corporate-run pharmacies—CVS, Rite Aid, Walgreens, and the local chain Duane Reade (which was soon bought by Walgreens)—were close friends of the tobacco companies, selling about 10 percent of the cigarettes in the city. I had three arguments in favor of banning cigarette sales there. First, pharmacies got a huge amount of foot traffic; it was wrong that smokers trying to quit should be tempted by power walls every time they bought medicine. Second, pharmacists are licensed health care professionals, like nurses and doctors; their selling cigarettes implied a tragic medical endorsement. Third, there was a weird and troubling conflict of interest in pharmacists selling cigarettes and then selling the antibiotics and inhalers to treat smoking-caused diseases.

I also proposed to prohibit sales of cigarettes within 500 feet of the city's middle and high schools. It seemed the most defensible way to cut the number of cigarette retailers. Nearly all smokers start as teenagers, and despite the law prohibiting sales to minors, nearly a third of high school kids in New York City who smoked said that they bought cigarettes from stores. Studies showed that teens living in neighborhoods with more stores selling cigarettes were more likely to smoke—maybe from the greater opportunity to buy cigarettes or maybe from the power walls' advertising. A sales ban near schools would least prevent kids from buying cigarettes or seeing ads when they dropped into bodegas during their lunch breaks. A 500-foot tobacco-free buffer around schools would cut the number of cigarette sellers by about 1,900—or 16 percent—which we would phase out when their two-year licenses came up for renewal.

The mayor was intrigued but skeptical. He felt that government had a duty to protect its citizens' health, but he was also a wildly successful businessman who bristled at government interference with private enterprise. My ideas straddled the fault line of those beliefs. He thought the sales buffer around schools would be overreaching—the government already banned sales of cigarettes to children under age eighteen, and he didn't accept the argument that the power walls themselves caused kids to smoke. The pharmacy ban also troubled him. What would be the financial impact on pharmacies? Were there any other examples of legal products that only certain businesses weren't allowed to sell? And would the sales ban really make any difference in smoking rates?

In the same meeting, I floated a third idea. The summer before, I had fumbled a press event and—without clearing it with City Hall—put a story on the front page of the *Times* endorsing a ban on smoking in parks and on beaches. We killed the story until after the election, but now I proposed to resurrect it. Of all of the expansions of the Smoke-Free Air Act that Perl had considered, this one looked the easiest to defend.

In the seven years since Frieden's round table advisers had told him not to do it, hundreds of cities and towns—including Los Angeles, San Francisco, and Chicago—had banned smoking in parks. Maintenance workers at New York's Department of Parks and Recreation hated the littered cigarette butts, especially on the beaches, where they stubbornly slipped through the prongs of the litter rakes. A San Francisco study showed that 25 percent of litter items on beaches came from cigarettes. People don't want their beaches to be ashtrays, I told Bloomberg. As the city's doctor, I wanted to make smoking even more socially unacceptable—to "denormalize" it. When a parent takes a young child to the park to kick a soccer ball, I said, that child shouldn't be getting a lesson in how to smoke.

But I suspected that Bloomberg's decision would turn on how much exposure to secondhand smoke people actually got outdoors. It wasn't a lot, but it wasn't zero either. The clearest study we found showed that someone within three feet of a smoker outdoors, depending on how the wind was blowing, could be breathing levels of secondhand smoke that were similar to those found around smokers indoors.

Bloomberg wasn't convinced. He understood that cigarettes bred litter, but people threw food wrappers on the ground too, and we weren't banning eating in parks. He rejected the "denormalizing" reason. If we banned behavior just because the spectacle offended some people, where would that stop? The city's ultra-Orthodox Jews were offended seeing women in bathing suits. And he was dubious about the risk of secondhand smoke outdoors. Was the exposure really enough to matter? I acknowledged that the risk was low, but tried this analogy: secondhand smoke is more carcinogenic than benzene. If we were to discover that benzene helped the grass grow, would we allow the parks department to spray it on the lawns, saying, "Don't worry, it might cause cancer in only a few people a year"?

In the end, the mayor approved only the proposal on parks and beaches. Although he could have enforced the smoke-free policy as a parks department rule, he agreed to propose it as a city law in a nod to the Speaker Christine Quinn, who liked the idea and wanted to take it through the City Council.

. . .

Just before that meeting, the tobacco companies fired their salvo against the in-store warning signs. Anne Pearson needn't have worried that they weren't taking the issue seriously. Indeed, they hated it. The suit rode in on a battalion of lawyers, as each of the big three tobacco companies bankrolled its own firm—Greenberg Traurig for Lorillard; Gibson, Dunn & Crutcher for Philip Morris; and Jones Day for R.J. Reynolds. Another firm—Cahill, Gordon & Reindel—represented the convenience stores. At the head of this army stood celebrity First Amendment lawyer Floyd Abrams, who was also representing the tobacco companies against the FDA's rule to put graphic warnings on cigarette packs. The companies argued that the warning signs were preempted by federal law that governed labeling of cigarette packs. They said the rule trampled on their First Amendment guarantee of free speech. And because of the Constitution's separation of powers, the Board of Health didn't have the authority to write the rule in the first place. Our attempt to warn people to avoid a drug that killed one-third of its users, in their considered view, threatened the very foundations of our democracy.

12

"We were outgunned."

Throughout the 2000s, obesity continued to swell as a slow-moving crisis. By 2008, 3.4 million of the city's 6 million adults were overweight or obese, and more than half a million had diabetes. Although no one is labeled as having died from excess body fat, the health department's epidemiologists estimated that the obesity in the city was responsible for at least 5,000 deaths a year. That was not as many as were killed by smoking, but it was close. Imagine the panic in the streets, I thought, if a virus were killing that many people.

Despite our efforts, we had no reason to think we were changing what New Yorkers ate. Not long after I started, Lynn Silver's team was wrapping up an evaluation of the calorie labeling on restaurant menu boards. Before and after the labels went up, her group had surveyed more than 11,000 customers as they exited 275 locations of the city's thirteen biggest chains. They found big increases in the proportion of people who noticed the calorie labels (from 11 to 56 percent) and in those who said they used them (from 3 to 15 percent), but mixed results on what people actually bought. In four chains—McDonald's, KFC, Starbucks, and Au Bon Pain—people walked away with 20 to 80 fewer calories in their food. In several chains the calories they purchased didn't change.

But in one chain—Subway—the number of calories purchased increased. Subway was unique. Even before the law went into effect, the chain had voluntarily put stickers with calorie counts on its display cases. And then in between the two data-collection waves, Subway had unleashed its "$5 footlong" sandwich promotion. Between the two surveys, the proportion of customers who bought twelve-inch sandwiches jumped from 28 to 73 percent.

Shortly after Silver showed these results at a scientific meeting, a group of economists published a study using data from the computerized cash registers at Starbucks. Customers at the coffee chain typically didn't buy a lot of calories; still, the researchers found that after the calorie labels went up, the customers bought 14 percent fewer. Because they had data on all the transactions, the researchers could also answer a crucial question that we couldn't: Starbucks did not see any fall in its sales overall. Its customers spent the same money on lower-caloric foods and drinks. So the calorie counts were helping some people buy fewer calories, but the effect was small, varied by chain, and could be overwhelmed if the restaurants marketed unhealthy foods aggressively.

After the years of painstaking work designing the calorie-label rule and the battle scars from two lawsuits, we found that conclusion disappointing. We all still believed that the labels were worth spreading nationally. The numbers helped some people, they raised red flags over particularly hefty foods, and maybe over time they would shame the restaurants into shrinking their giant items, or at least slowing the portion arms race. But on their own they weren't going to make a dent in the obesity epidemic. We needed better solutions. For Lynn Silver, the studies "highlighted that we had to go beyond information interventions probably into actual regulation of the practices of restaurants."

In 2009 we didn't have specific ideas on regulating restaurants, so we came back to sugary drinks. We had hopes for taking a second swing at a soda tax. And soon after I started, Geoff Cowley wanted to show me some counter-ads that had grown out of Mary Bassett's junk food group.

When we had first tried to rally support for a sugary drink tax in neighborhoods that were hard hit by obesity, we had met stiff resistance. Everyone knew that French fries and cupcakes made you fat, but soda? People didn't see sugary drinks as a health problem, so they saw a soda tax as just government greed. When we first contemplated sugary drink counter-ads, we meant them to persuade people to drink less soda. Now that the tax idea was in the air, though, we realized that ads might build political support for it, too.

In coming up with good counter-ads, we faced a problem with deep roots. Like cigarettes, soda isn't just sold—it's marketed. Its brilliant advertising, about $1 billion a year in Coke polar bears and Pepsi pop stars, overwhelms our televisions, sports stadiums, movie theaters, delis, bodegas, pizza joints, and snack counters. Coke and Pepsi reinforce those powerful ads by inserting their sodas into movies and TV shows and by sponsoring museums, parks, sports teams, and the Olympics. They put bottles in Americans' hands with all of the other P's of marketing: clever packaging, tempting prices, and in-your-face placement.

The marketing that Americans have been subjected to—over generations—has welded an intense emotional attachment to the Coke and Pepsi brands. When a father takes his son on his sixth birthday to see his first Major League baseball game and buys the boy a hot dog and a Coke, it creates a golden memory. For the rest of that boy's life, when he wants a little emotional lift, he will grab a Coke. The marketing geniuses in Atlanta know that and have been playing variations on that theme for a century. Coke is Santa Claus, Coke is happiness, Coke is America. And Pepsi is youth, fun, and excitement. To tell New Yorkers that Coke and Pepsi meant blubber and diabetes would provoke ugly emotions.

Jeffrey Escoffier had ordered up some anti-sugary-drink ads from Jose Bandujo, who ran an advertising agency that was on contract with the department. "Don't worry if it's tasteful or anything," he later remembered telling Bandujo. "Just do whatever you can so that it's strong and a hard-hitting thing on soda." Then Escoffier tested them with focus groups of soda drinkers, some of whom were overweight.

The problem we faced showed up immediately. In the warm-up, the participants commented that they didn't think of sugary drinks as healthy, but they didn't see them as truly unhealthy either. "Anything in moderation is okay," said one woman. Yeah, said another, drinking one or two sodas a day wasn't a problem. In fact, an additional one or two sodas every day might be enough to drive the entire obesity epidemic.

The moderator passed around several sets of ads, face down, then asked the participants to turn them over one set a time. One pair of ads made our problem even clearer. The images showed morbidly obese men in stained T-shirts, guzzling soda from 2-liter bottles, and the text said that soda "just dumps sugar and calories into your system. This can lead to obesity, high blood pressure, and diabetes." The participants refused to believe it. Bandujo remembered, "Immediately people said, 'He didn't get that fat from just soda. He got fat from McDonald's. He got fat from fast food. He got fat from other stuff.'" They were also convinced that people as fat as those in the ads must just have "bad genes."

Other ads proved that we were in treacherous emotional waters. One set mocked soda brands, showing glasses or bottles labeled "Dr. Diabetes" and "Mountain Don't." The participants were offended on behalf of the soda companies. "It was like we were talking bad about their mother," said Beth Kilgore. "And they even got their legal hat on," said Bandujo. "'Oh, are you allowed to do that?' Poor Mountain Dew!"

Another group of ads mixed a tough message with a touch of humor. A woman's huge buttocks were labeled "Soda Can." A guy's gut (going after "sports drinks") was branded "Sports Section."

When a group of women turned over the pictures, there was a flutter of nervous laughter. "That's what *my* stomach looks like." "I'm like, wow, *I* could look like this." "This is *really* offensive because it is real."

One ad from this group showed a little girl's fat stomach pushing out her bathing suit, with the label "Juice Container." This one was too painful even to laugh at. "I felt sorry for her," one man said sadly. "It's cruel to show kids."

We couldn't run ads like those. Even if they worked, they would spark a firestorm among overweight New Yorkers and light up the tabloids.

Bandujo's team had come up with another idea, one that went directly at people's disbelief. "People could easily rationalize in their head that when you eat a cupcake, it turns to fat," he said. "When you eat a hot dog, it turns to fat. . . . People weren't thinking of a liquid turning into a solid—fat!" The ad just showed a can of soda being poured into a glass, but as the soda fell, it turned into yellowish globules of fat laced with thin red blood vessels. In big letters beneath, the ad asked "Are you pouring on the pounds?"

Among women, the ad worked beautifully. One said, "I can't even look at this." Another said, "It has my stomach churning." She thought she might vomit right then. Another said, "I would put it on my refrigerator" to remind her not to drink soda. But the men shrugged; to them, the fat globules weren't disgusting enough. One man said helpfully, "Maybe if you showed somebody *drinking* it . . ."

Still, "revulsion was the most effective approach," the focus group summary report read. "What we've learned in public health is that negative is very good," said Bandujo. "Negative is what makes them think."

I liked the soda-turning-into-fat ads instantly and got approval to run them. We posted three versions on the subways showing different beverages: a cola (in a plastic bottle with a red label), a lime green sports drink (in a plastic bottle with an orange cap), and an iced tea (in a glass bottle with a yellow label). None of them had any brand names or logos. The headline "ARE YOU POURING ON THE POUNDS?" was now followed by "Don't drink yourself fat. Cut back on soda and other sugary beverages. Go with water, seltzer, or low-fat milk instead."

The subway ads stirred up just the kind of chatter that we wanted. The *Times* story said that the health department had "opened a new front in their struggle against high-calorie beverages." Their editors wrote, "The city's health department has gone the yuck route, which officials say worked well with cigarette ads. . . . Smoking in the city went down after television commercials showed a man with a hole in his throat and a woman with missing fingers." The American Beverage Association, calling the campaign "over the top," tried to divert attention to everything else. The ads would "undermine meaningful efforts to educate people about how to maintain a healthy weight by balancing calories consumed from all foods and beverages with calories burned through exercise."

But Jose Bandujo wasn't finished. That focus group participant's suggestion had given him an idea. He and a producer hired an acting student, sent colleagues to the grocery store to buy the "grossest stuff we could think of to make this yellowish orange-ish chunky concoction," and turned on their video cameras. In the video, backed up by campy music, the actor pops open a can of soda to pour it into a glass, but what plops into the glass is globules of fat. Then the actor tips up the glass and gulps it down, the fat blobs overflowing onto his cheeks and down his chin. Words drop onto the screen to the sounds of deep echoing booms: "DON'T DRINK YOURSELF FAT." Then, holding up the glass of fat as if to propose a toast, the young man turns to the camera, smiles, and gives a mischievous wink.

When I saw it, I burst out laughing. Our cigarette ads had needed a dead-serious tone. But people weren't fully ready to hear that sugary drinks made you sick. This ad managed to deliver that tough message with a smirk and a punch line. I couldn't wait to release it.

But then we got stuck on the words that would appear on the screen. At first, they were "Drinking a can of soda is like drinking 150 calories of fat." We couldn't say that, I told my staff. The problem with soda was the sugar, and metabolically, sugar *wasn't* like fat. Eating a giant blob of fat was bad for you, but in a different way. The point about sugary drinks, I insisted, was not that they were *like* fat but that they *made you* fat. The words had to be about weight gain. But how much weight? After a few days of haggling with my team over e-mail about the tagline, I settled on a number and included a flexible word, ending up with "Drinking 1 can of soda a day . . . can make you 10 pounds fatter a year." I also suggested adding a small disclaimer like "assuming no other changes in diet or physical activity." But my staff never added the disclaimer, and I didn't notice that they hadn't.

We had no money to run the ad on television, so we just posted *Man Drinking Fat* on YouTube and sent out a press release. The ad incited a swarm of outraged "sharing." "The best thing you can do on a viral video is to get some comments like 'This is the grossest thing ever,'" said Bandujo. "Everybody needs to click on that to see what it is." In its first week online, *Man Drinking Fat* got nearly a half million views and a piece of Jay Leno's monologue. With all the outrage, the ad was doing exactly what we wanted—getting people to talk about how sugary drinks make you fat.

. . .

After we got past the election, I met with Mayor Bloomberg to propose a new push for a soda tax. I had heard that the Greater New York Hospital Association and the hospital workers' union were planning to lobby hard for a soda tax in the next legislative session, and I wanted to put the city's political power behind it. By then we had new estimates from an academic expert that a 1-cent-per-ounce tax might reduce sales by 8 percent, stop 60,000 people in New York City from becoming obese, and prevent 7,500 from developing diabetes.

As a businessman, Bloomberg instinctively believed that raising the price was the surest way to cut sales of anything. With the state still in a budget crisis, the legislature would be hungry for money. He thought we should present a simple trade-off: we could have a soda tax that generated a billion dollars a year and save the jobs of thousands of teachers or cops, or we could skip the tax and lay them off.

In January 2010, Governor David Paterson did propose another soda tax, along with a dollar-per-pack increase in the state cigarette tax, as part of a package to fill the state's projected deficit of $7.4 billion. Even with the soda tax and the higher cigarette tax, the governor proposed big spending cuts, slashing $1.1 billion in funding for schools and $900 million in payments to hospitals, nursing homes, and home care agencies.

This time the governor got the soda tax right. His new proposal was a 1-cent-per-ounce excise tax, with the revenue paying for health care. The sugary drink distributors would pay the tax based on how much they shipped. Everyone assumed—from experience with cigarette taxes—that the distributors would pass the cost on to retailers, who would then raise the prices for sugary drinks at stores and restaurants. The proposal was much better than Paterson's sales tax idea the year before. The tax would be simpler to collect because there weren't many distributors in the state. Because it would increase the price seen by consumers, the tax would cut sales more. The tax would grow as the volume of soda grew, encouraging people to buy less. Channeling the tax revenue to health care would help get voters behind it. One poll found that while only 47 percent of voters supported an "obesity tax," 76 percent supported "a tax on sugary soft drinks to balance the city budget." In a second poll, 76 percent preferred a soda tax to cuts in health care.

A week later Bloomberg jumped on board. He said to the legislature, "Today, more than half the residents of New York City, and nearly forty percent of our public school students, are overweight," which put them "dangerously on track to contracting diabetes" and other health problems. So "it's in the interest of us all to prevent that from happening now—and the surest pathway to changing behavior is through the wallet."

The year before we had been caught off guard, but this time we thought we had a good chance of passing the tax. All pulling in the same direction were the governor, the mayor, the hospitals, the union of hospital workers, and a charged-up coalition of health organizations, including the American Heart Association, the American Cancer Society, and the American Diabetes Association. Each played a part. State health commissioner Richard Daines wrote op-eds, met with editorial boards, and barnstormed the state, haranguing anyone willing to listen about the soda tax's "triple play": better health, less need for treatment, more money for health care. The hospitals were among the biggest employers in the state, and their 1199 SEIU union supported political campaigns, so they both had clout. Together with the health advocacy coalition, they put in more than 7,000 phone calls to legislators, met with more than a hundred of them, held a rally with 250 health care workers at the capitol, and held symbolic "soda buy-back" events around the state. They also ran television ads that featured doctors and nutritionists talking about the damage obesity was causing in kids and the link to sugary drinks. "It's an epidemic, and it's preventable," one nutritionist says. "It's a matter of life and death if action is not taken," says another. The ad ends, "Tell Albany to pass the soda tax. Make New York healthier."

Paterson's tax proposal the year before had caught the soda companies by surprise, too. But they had recovered quickly, spending the time between legislative sessions trying to strangle the idea. In September 2009, Coke and its largest bottler said they were running advertising campaigns in seven key markets to kill soda tax proposals. "Clearly, the threat of a soft drink tax demonstrates the need to better educate our consumers on what we're doing to be part of the solution to the obesity problem," a spokeswoman said. Ten days later an op-ed appeared in *The Wall Street Journal* under the byline Muhtar Kent, the CEO of Coca-Cola. He argued that sugary drinks accounted for only 5.5 percent of calories in the average American diet, that obesity is "also about calories out," and that a soda tax would hurt the poor without changing people's soda habits. Soon afterward we noticed ads appearing from Coke under the slogan "Live positively," in which they touted how they were "doing our part" to fight obesity with "portion control options, choice, and innovation."

When Paterson proposed the new tax, the soda companies turned for help in the battle to Goddard Claussen, the "issue advocacy" public relations company behind the "Harry and Louise" ad had that helped kill Bill Clinton's health care reform plan. Under its new name Goddard Gunster, the agency today calls itself "the most sought-after guns for hire," which is proud to be "among the first to apply aggressive political campaign strategies to issue advocacy efforts." Its website explains its technique: "Through facts and research, we define the parameters of the public debate and align consumer, corporate, and government interests."

Goddard Claussen created an Astroturf group called New Yorkers Against Unfair Taxes and fired back with an ad campaign of its own. One ad featured a Bronx grocer calling the soda tax "just another way to get into our pockets." "They talk about a penny here, a penny there, but you know what? In our type of community, it all adds up. . . . New Yorkers cannot afford another tax." In another, a woman unloading groceries tells the viewer, "Making ends meet is a constant struggle for families like ours. . . . Instead of cutting out-of-control spending in Albany, [Governor Paterson would] tax families. . . . Tell Albany to trim their budget fat, and leave our grocery budgets alone."

The ads, though, were just the visible part of the battle. The serious combat took place in back rooms. In 2009, after the first soda tax proposals in New York State and then in Washington, Coke, Pepsi, and the American Beverage Association increased their federal lobbying spending eightfold, from $4.7 to $40.3 million. In New York State in 2009, the

ABA increased its donations to state legislators from nothing to $900,000, and the two soda companies increased their state lobbying spending to $3 million. That included $36,000 that was channeled to State Senator Jeff Klein, who then switched from being a soda tax supporter to one who was, according to an inside source for the *Daily News*, "instrumental in getting the soda tax off the table."

After Paterson's 2010 proposal, Coke and Pepsi sent workers to meet with the governor. The tax would kill their jobs, they told him. The companies also claimed that as they passed on the cost of tax to customers, they couldn't create a price difference between sugary drinks and diet drinks, which would defeat the tax's obesity-prevention purpose. They brought in the Teamsters, whose members drive soda delivery trucks, to pressure union-friendly legislators. To make sure those legislators heeded their arguments, the ABA opened its wallet further, spending nearly $13 million, which put it atop the list of lobbyists for any issue in 2010. And as part of a behind-the-scenes charm offensive, both Coke's CEO Muhtar Kent and PepsiCo's CEO Indra Nooyi contacted Bloomberg, offering to work with us on pilot projects in the city.

The legislators in Albany listened. In March 2010, about six weeks after Paterson released his budget, I drove to the capitol and met with several representatives, to whom I handed out one-pagers with facts on the obesity crisis and the benefits of a soda tax. The legislators were cordial, but all except for a few were dead set against it. When I spoke to State Senator Ruth Hassell-Thompson, a nurse who was otherwise strong on health issues, she cut me off. There was no way she could support the tax, she said. I knew that PepsiCo's headquarters was not far from her district in Westchester County. Dean Skelos, the ranking Republican senator, listened politely but asked rhetorically, "When has a tax ever changed behavior?" I wasn't quick enough to answer by talking about the cigarette tax. A week later all the state's Republican senators, and enough of the chamber's Democrats to form a majority, were publicly opposed to the tax.

By May, Paterson was flailing. He suggested exempting diet soda from the state's sales tax in return for keeping his soda tax. Then state health commissioner Richard Daines called me to suggest the tax apply in New York City only, with all the revenue flowing to the state government and none going to the city. Neither idea made headway.

By July, reporters were writing postmortems. The soda tax "was pretty much a nonstarter, politically," said Deputy Mayor Howard Wolfson later. Wolfson, who had run communications for Hillary Clinton's 2008 presidential campaign, was now the mayor's top adviser on political strategy and communications. In his conversations with legislators, the idea was "DOA. Not gonna happen." Michael Nutter, the mayor of Philadelphia who had himself failed to pass a 2-cents-an-ounce soda tax, summed up the soda company tactics: "They're successful the old-fashioned way. They pay for it." "We were outgunned," said the political director of the hospital workers' union. Coke and Pepsi had shown that they were stronger than a governor, a mayor, and the state's health commissioners, hospitals, and most powerful union combined.

The failure of the tax certainly wasn't caused by the legislature being antitax or concerned with the impact on the poor. Although the soda companies said the legislators killed the soda tax because it was regressive, the lawmakers instead passed a 4 percent sales tax on clothing, which was far less fair: people have to buy clothes, but they don't have to buy soda. At the same time, without any pressure from health groups that I know of, the legislators took Paterson's dollar-per-pack cigarette tax increase proposal 60 cents further, increasing the total state tax on a pack of cigarettes from $2.75 to $4.35. With the federal tax of $1.01 and the city's tax of $1.50 per pack, the total tax on a pack of cigarettes sold in New York City was now $6.86, bringing the price to about $11, the highest in the nation. The shot we had fired at soda landed on cigarettes instead.

13

"Would you like us to say, 'That's not our responsibility'?"

In April 2010 we were finally ready to announce the names of companies that had promised to cut the amount of salt they put in food. It had been three years since Mary Bassett, Lynn Silver, and Sonia Angell had first presented the idea to Tom Frieden, and eighteen months since the Salt Summit at Gracie Mansion. During that time, their team had built momentum with health organizations. What we now called the National Salt Reduction Initiative (NSRI) stretched across the country, boasting six city health departments, fifteen state health departments, and seventeen national organizations, including the American Medical Association, the American Heart Association, and Consumers Union.

The nation's food companies weren't so enthusiastic. In the months since the Salt Summit, Angell and Christine Curtis had held more than one hundred meetings with the food giants. The companies complained that the targets were too stringent, the deadlines too near, the technical problems too overwhelming, and the customers too wedded to the salty taste. Technical experts at some companies told our staff privately that the targets were not hard to hit, even as other representatives were complain-

161

ing how tough they were. But so far it had all been vague talk. Until the commitments came in, we had no idea whether most of the U.S. food industry would sign on or ignore us.

We had released the targets three months earlier. They applied to sixty-one packaged-food categories, including "French toast, pancakes, and waffles," "Frozen and refrigerated meat substitutes," processed cheese, "Salsa, dips, and dipping sauce," "Frozen and refrigerated pizza," canned soup, and crackers. After haggling, ketchup was now embedded in "Barbecue sauce, ketchup, marinades, and steak sauce." The restaurants had targets for twenty-five categories, including hamburgers, cheeseburgers, sandwiches, burritos, and French fries. Each category had an easier target for 2012 and a stricter one for 2014. The 2014 targets would cut salt by an average of 25 percent, but the cuts in the different food categories ranged from 10 to 35 percent.

Once we circulated those targets, the press had a chance to size up the initiative. Despite the fears of Bloomberg's press officer Stu Loeser, the papers liked the plan. The *Daily News* featured a medical assistant from Brooklyn whose diet of bacon-and-egg sandwiches, ham sandwiches, hot dogs, and chicken nuggets fed her more than three times the recommendations. The *Times* put the story on the front page, calling salt a "health scourge." But the "campaign is in some ways more ambitious and less certain of success than the ones it waged against smoking and obesity. . . . For one thing, the changes it prescribes require cooperation on a national scale." *The Wall Street Journal* wrote, "Decreasing salt is one of the thorniest challenges in food science," and quoted a food scientist saying that salt replacements were "never cheaper than sodium chloride, unfortunately."

When reporters asked Bloomberg if taking on salt was overreaching, he snapped, "We're not controlling how much salt [people eat]. . . . We're trying to extend the lives and improve the lives of people that live in this City. And the health department has that responsibility. Would you like us to stop if there was asbestos in the air in your building or in the place your child goes to school? Would you like us to say, 'That's not our responsibility'? I don't think so."

The *Times*'s personal health columnist Jane Brody wrote a glowing piece. "If the mayor has his way," she wrote, "this could well be the year when salt, once a form of legal tender, is finally devalued as a prized condiment in the American diet." She cited a well-timed study estimating that a half-teaspoon less salt intake per day would save 44,000 to 92,000 lives a year. "That, dear reader, would be a very big bang for a relatively small buck."

When Sylvia Birnbaum, the woman who failed to escape hypertension, heard about the initiative, she thought it was a great idea. But she asked a poignant question: "Why haven't they thought about that years ago?" It seems she wasn't alone. A month later, when the Quinnipiac Polling Institute asked New Yorkers, "Do you think the Bloomberg administration is correct to encourage New York City restaurants to use less salt in food preparation?," 77 percent said yes. And when it asked, "When it comes to trying to improve people's health habits, do you think the Bloomberg administration's policies have gone too far, not far enough, or they are about right?," 55 percent said "about right" and another 17 percent said "not far enough." "There's been some grumbling about 'nanny government' by Mayor Michael Bloomberg," Quinnipiac's polling director said, "but voters are eating it up. . . . City Hall's menu of food initiatives gets three stars from voters."

But the food industry pushed back, and the federal government seemed to be wilting. The Grocery Manufacturers Association issued familiar complaints about the NSRI. Cutting sodium would run into "regulatory, human capital, and technical barriers" and would alter "taste, texture, appearance, shelf-life, or price" in a way that "may not be acceptable to consumers." And the initiative should be led by the federal government, not by New York City. The National Restaurant Association was even more abrupt. It was simply "opposed to a Federal, state, or local mandate on specific nutrients or ingredients."

At first, we had hoped to get the FDA and the CDC to endorse the National Salt Reduction Initiative. Then FDA staff said an endorsement of a voluntary initiative wouldn't be "appropriate" for a regulatory agency. We asked instead for supportive statements from the two agencies to fold into our press release. That didn't happen either. Finally, the

CDC issued its own feeble statement that it "supports efforts to reduce the sodium content of manufactured and restaurant foods," without mentioning the NSRI by name. Someone high up in the federal government, I figured, someone above Tom Frieden and above the FDA, must be stonewalling.

A month after we released the targets, Michael Alderman, a doctor who served for many years on an advisory committee to the industry's Salt Institute, published an opinion piece in the *Journal of the American Medical Association*. The studies on salt didn't meet the standard of proof, he claimed. Cutting salt levels in food was a "rash route" that might actually increase deaths. We needed massive, multiyear studies, and in the meantime "the prudent course of action may well be caution." It was a well-worn argument for paralysis. *JAMA*'s publishing it, unfortunately, gave it legitimacy.

• • •

We planned a splashy announcement to recognize the companies that pledged to meet our salt targets. As the event approached, the positive signals coming from the companies surprised us. Mars, a company with $7 billion in sales that was best known for its candy bars but that also makes Uncle Ben's rice mixes, said it planned to sign on. Then three food giants made statements that sounded like real action. In March, Kraft Foods, a behemoth that sold $24 billion in food across twenty-three of our categories, from Oscar Mayer cold cuts to Philadelphia Cream Cheese, announced it would be cutting sodium by an average of 10 percent for all its North American products by 2012. That same month PepsiCo, which owned Frito-Lay and Quaker and had even more food sales than Kraft, declared that it would cut its average salt levels by 25 percent by 2015. Staff from both companies told us privately that we could expect letters committing to meet at least some of our salt targets. Unilever, a conglomerate making Wishbone salad dressing and Ragú pasta sauces, had already announced in 2009 that it was cutting salt in all 22,000 of its products. Now Unilever was telling us that it would meet several of our targets. And we even got word that some huge restaurant chains (including Subway and Starbucks) would sign on. I was so excited that I e-mailed Angell and Silver to say, "We're changing the world!"

For a moment, it even looked as if we might get the federal government to support the NSRI indirectly. Three agencies involved in nutrition—the CDC, the FDA, and the U.S. Department of Agriculture—were planning a Nutrition Summit in April entitled "Changing the Food Environment." The conference objectives were so ambitious for the federal government that they could only have been written by Tom Frieden. They included promoting restaurant menu calorie labeling, reducing trans fats, and cutting salt levels in processed foods. We were negotiating to insert Mayor Bloomberg into the event for our announcement thanking the companies that promised to cut salt in their foods. That would not only give the companies even more good press but also imply that the big three federal agencies were in favor of what we were doing.

But then, over just a few days, everything seemed to unravel. First, the big companies backed off. They claimed different reasons. Kraft's lawyers were balking at the word *commitment,* Sonia Angell heard. PepsiCo wouldn't jump in, Lynn Silver heard, unless it saw a commitment from at least one of the other big food companies—which it saw as ConAgra, Kraft, Unilever, and Campbell Soup. An employee of Unilever said that before promising anything, his company wanted to see an impending report on salt from the respected Institute of Medicine (IOM). We heard that the real obstacle was the Grocery Manufacturers Association, which was pressuring the companies to close ranks against us.

Then the IOM ran away with the conversation. In 2008 Congress had asked it to develop recommendations for reducing sodium in the American diet. Angell was one of the fourteen members on the IOM committee, which was chaired by former FDA commissioner Jane Henney. Days before we were scheduled to announce our companies' salt pledges, the committee issued an uncompromising report: it recommended that the FDA "set mandatory national standards" for salt consumption. Over the long term, the committee wrote, voluntary initiatives like ours were bound to fail. "There needs to be a mandatory standard," Dr. Henney told the Associated Press. "[H]aving one or two in the industry make strong attempts at this doesn't give us that even playing field over time. It's not sustainable."

Just as the IOM announced this pointed conclusion, *The Washington Post* ran a front-page story, quoting anonymous sources within the FDA, headlined "FDA READYING FIRST LEGAL LIMITS ON AMOUNT OF SALT IN FOODS." Immediately Senator Tom Harkin and Representative Rosa DeLauro heartily endorsed the FDA's regulating salt. To anyone reading the papers, it looked as if the federal government were going to force food companies to use less salt, and do so very soon.

I would have been overjoyed if the FDA were set to regulate salt, but I knew it wasn't going to happen. The FDA is too much under the thumb of the food corporations' friends in Congress. Even when the agency does move, it takes years. And sure enough, the next day the FDA issued a statement calling the *Post* "mistaken." "The FDA is not currently working on regulation nor have we made a decision to regulate sodium content of food at this time." Still, I was worried that all this blunt talk about mandates and regulation might make the food companies hunker down instead of work with us.

Then our hope for federal endorsement at the Nutrition Summit fell apart. The summit's objectives were watered down—conference organizers told us that no new policies were going to be announced there. CDC staff told us that Bloomberg was welcome to make his announcement at their conference, but they would make clear that it was "a NYC event not a federal or summit event." Furthermore, the CDC and the FDA wouldn't make even vaguely supportive statements about our initiative. The FDA wouldn't send a representative to our announcement, and although the CDC might send one, she would not say a word. Now that we were poised to accomplish something that the federal health agencies had been recommending for decades, those agencies were running and hiding. It was so sad that it was almost comical.

In what looked like the final blow, City Hall press officer Stu Loeser threatened to cancel Bloomberg's announcement itself. The federal government seemed to be stealing the narrative, he thought, after seeing the stories on the FDA. Besides, Loeser had offered the story to a reporter at

The Wall Street Journal as an exclusive, and the reporter was unimpressed. Companies saying they would reduce their "sales-weighted average" sodium level for crackers to 640 mg per 100 grams would mean nothing to readers. The reporter needed to see changes to specific, recognizable products for them to feel real. "There's no story here," a press staffer told us.

The companies were dropping out, the federal agencies were melting away, and the event itself was evaporating. In a few days, we had gone from changing the world to looking hopelessly inept.

The salt team met in my office in despair. Should we drop the whole effort and declare failure? But Lynn Silver, Sonia Angell, and Christine Curtis had worked for years for this moment. They had created forward movement out of little but chutzpah, data, and persistence. After decades in which the federal health agencies had accomplished zero on salt, the New York City health department had actually prodded the massive food industry to budge.

We rallied to hold it together. Heinz had promised to cut the sodium in its ketchup by 15 percent by 2012. That achievement, as small as it seemed, was heartening to my chief of staff, Kelly Christ. Heinz ketchup was as big and as American as any food gets. Her five-year-old niece ate Heinz ketchup every single day, like "every toddler in America." Cutting how much salt we were feeding those kids was damned important. And there couldn't be a more concrete example for the *Journal*. With some frantic calling, the group uncovered a few examples of specific foods that would lose some salt. They weren't thrilling—Oscar Meyer bologna down 17 percent, Goya canned beans down 25 percent—but they were just enough to satisfy the reporter.

I lobbied Stu Loeser and Linda Gibbs. Federal regulation at this point was a pipe dream; the FDA story was a distraction. Mayor Bloomberg was often accused of liking heavy-handed government regulations; this was a chance to show him cooperating with industry. He had created the salt story and he deserved to get the credit for it. And if we canceled the announcement, we'd be fighting ugly stories about why our well-publicized initiative had flopped. That got the event back on the mayor's calendar.

On a Monday afternoon, Bloomberg led a small entourage into City Hall's Blue Room. I stood behind him, together with American Heart Association CEO Nancy Brown, Los Angeles health director Jonathan Fielding, and representatives from Mars, Subway, and other food companies. "Now I must make an admission here," the mayor started. "I love salt on my food. I'll put it on my popcorn. I'll put it on my bagels. I'll even sprinkle it on my saltines." Having gotten that out of the way, he went on. "Today I'm excited to announce that sixteen of those companies have formally committed to our National Salt Reduction Initiative. . . . In total, these companies have made commitments to reduce sodium in 49 of the 62 packaged food categories and 15 of the 25 restaurant food categories. . . . They are true leaders in their industry."

Those companies that had taken the leap were promising some important changes. Boar's Head, a sandwich meat maker, committed to meeting 2014 targets in cold cuts, sausage, bacon, and processed cheese. Starbucks promised to meet the standards for its breakfast sandwiches, Subway for its sandwiches, soup, and cookies, and Unilever for its pasta sauces. The grocery store distributor White Rose would require its private-label manufacturers to fall in line with targets for thirty-nine packaged food categories. And giant Kraft made a commitment that was frustratingly vague but potentially huge: it promised to "meet or exceed the sodium reduction targets in 50 percent of the relevant NSRI categories, which represents the large majority of the foods that we sell."

Many companies ignored us. PepsiCo, General Mills, and ConAgra were missing, as were McDonald's, Burger King, and Wendy's. Campbell Soup put out a statement that could have spoken for all those on the sidelines: "we believe the targets and timing proposed by New York City can not be realistically achieved in all of our product categories and still meet consumers' demand for great-tasting foods." Still, for the first time ever, America now had a concrete national plan to reduce the amount of salt in food. Many food companies were signing on, and if the rest of the food industry later joined them, every year tens of thousands fewer Americans would die of heart disease or stroke.

At the health department, we didn't know if our initiative would build momentum over time or stall. But we saw no alternative. The food companies hated mandates and wanted to be left alone on salt, but that hands-off approach had failed for decades. The Institute of Medicine committee wanted mandatory regulation, but only the FDA could do that, and it looked paralyzed. Our scheme of coordinated and verified but voluntary action was an attempt at a middle path between two extremes that each looked like dead ends.

. . .

A few days after I landed as health commissioner in 2009, Farzad Mostashari came to my office and told me he was leaving. He was headed to the federal government as a deputy to David Blumenthal, the national coordinator for health information technology. When Mostashari left, I asked Amanda Parsons, from his unit, to take over New York City's Primary Care Information Project.

Parsons is not a typical doctor or a typical Frieden disciple. Young, blond, and effervescent, she had found her way to the health department not though the mountains of Nicaragua but through the sleek offices of the Fortune 500. Beside her M.D., she had an M.B.A. and several years' experience advising drug companies for the consulting firm McKinsey & Company. By 2007, after Frieden's high-profile successes, even at McKinsey "people were *talking* about the health department." When a job announcement in Mostashari's electronic medical records project popped up, Parsons had sent in a résumé. As his new quality improvement director, she would create teams that would show doctors how to use electronic health records to practice medicine better.

She was starting from zero. "None of [the doctors] spent any time thinking about quality improvement," she said. "They had no foundation to do it." Worse, even doctors who had completed the training on eClinicalWorks were "completely under water" with the software. They especially struggled with their lifeblood—billing, which was a key function of eClinicalWorks. For doctors in small practices, getting paid is a nightmare, with or without software. "The level of craziness is far beyond what I ever understood," Mostashari told me. "The regulatory requirements are so heavy that the doctors are clickety-clickety-clicking all day long, having nothing to do with what's really clinical care."

Before Parsons could coax doctors to think about improving quality, she had to throw them a lifeline. She established a team that did nothing but help configure doctors' software and give them booster training, and a second team that helped straighten out billing morasses.

Only after she got past that was Parsons able to send in a third team to focus on the quality of care. The quality team showed doctors how to generate lists of patients needing preventive tests or treatments, just as Mostashari had shown the doctor in Harlem which of her patients needed flu shots. Later Parsons filtered the lists based on the kind of action needed: those patients who hadn't been tested (like for diabetes), those who had been diagnosed but were not prescribed medicines, and those who were supposed to be taking medicine but had not been to the doctor for a long time.

Parsons' staff also calculated the doctors' quality measures, like the percent of patients over sixty-five who had had a flu shot. At first the doctors were embarrassed that their quality indicators were bad. But after getting over their initial skepticism, like the doctor in Harlem, they wanted to improve. They ran lists, sent their patients letters, and tracked their progress with the software.

In 2009 the Obama administration's "stimulus package" allocated money for the program Health Information Technology for Economic and Clinical Health (HITECH). HITECH would distribute $2 billion to help doctors adopt electronic medical records and billions more if the doctors achieved "meaningful use" of "qualified, certified" software. For the government to certify the software, it had to have certain features, and for doctors to get the incentive payments, they had to use those features. The "meaningful use" features were based on what Mostashari had learned from the New York City project, like "clinical decision support systems," the ability to generate filtered patient lists, and built-in quality-of-care measures. Of the $2 billion, more than $600 million was designated for "regional extension centers" that would help doctors exchange their paper charts for the software. These extension centers would copy what the New York City health department had done; they had been Far-zad Mostashari's idea.

By the time Parsons began directing the program in the summer of 2010, the Primary Care Information Project was mushrooming. Unbelievably, the team had fulfilled Bloomberg's first promise that a thousand doctors would be using the city's software by the end of 2008, and it would soon deliver on his second promise of 2,500 doctors by the end of 2010. The health department became one of the new regional extension centers, receiving federal funds. With that designation, the project expanded to help doctors use not just eClinicalWorks but any electronic medical record software that met the new federal standards. The project soon reached into the offices of doctors treating three million people.

Later, I visited one of those offices. Dr. Frank Maselli leads Riverdale Family Practice, a group of ten family physicians in the Bronx. He has a tree trunk for a chest and a broad black beard, making him look more like a down lineman than a family doc, but he also has a warm smile and a knack for computers. Riverdale was one of the early practices to install the health department's software and try out its quality-improvement features. "I got my first dashboard," Dr. Maselli told me. "It was horrible. . . . Everything's all red." It hurt, because he and his partners took pride in their work. "It's not like you have bad doctors. It's just that you have so many things to do. . . . It's so hard to keep all the balls in the air." When he talked to his doctors about flu shots and helping smokers quit, they told him, "'You just gave me a list of twelve more things I have to do. When am I going to do them?' And we realized that we had to take that function away from the doctors and give it to other members of the staff."

Dr. Maselli trained his medical assistants to routinely check the electronic records and ask patients about important actions that were easy to overlook—not just flu shots and smoking but also mammograms and colon cancer screens and cholesterol tests. The medical assistants updated the software and then prompted the doctor to write a prescription or give a vaccine. After he reassigned this routine work, Riverdale's "dashboard" of quality measures improved "tremendously."

When I spoke to Dr. Maselli, I was amazed at how the software had become so central to his practice. He demonstrated the features, his large hands nearly covering a tiny laptop's keyboard. Alerts about high blood pressure popped up on the screen. A click gave the doctors suggestions for treatment. Another click sent prescriptions to a patient's pharmacy. Laboratory test results arrived electronically, routed automatically into individual patient records. An office quality manager printed lists of patients who were overdue for appointments, tests, or services and then used the software to contact them. Every month the health department e-mailed Dr. Maselli quality reports for each of his doctors, and every month he passed them around among the doctors so everyone saw all of them, and by peer pressure all were motivated to improve. "The [health department] program was just great," he said. "It's been a terrific success."

As an enthusiastic adopter, Dr. Maselli wasn't typical. Amanda Parsons needed to know whether, across an ever-widening footprint, the project was actually helping most doctors practice medicine better. One of her staffers, Sarah Shih, conducted a study to find out. Doctors in fifty-six offices had received an early version of the health department's software, before the reminder systems were built. Later the health department added the preventive-service reminders and other quality features to their machines. Shih measured how often the doctors in those practices did ten different tests and treatments, first before they got the reminders and then six months afterward. Because the doctors had had electronic medical records the entire time, the study would assess not whether computerized records improved care but instead whether the reminder systems—the virtual Tom Frieden standing at their shoulders—made a difference.

And they did. After they got the reminders, doctors increased by more than 10 percentage points the number of patients they screened for breast cancer, measured for obesity, or tested for diabetes. They were also more likely to ask patients about smoking, give flu shots, and control high blood pressure. In all, the doctors' performance improved in seven of the ten measures of quality of preventive care. And it was a large majority of the doctors who were improving, not just a few head-of-the-class types.

When I saw the results, I was astounded. Big medical practices with full-time managers had shown similar improvements with the smart use of software. But the improvements in New York City were in tiny practices, often storefronts with just one or two doctors who had no organization looking over their shoulders. The software had filled in their blind spot. And with that new vision, the doctors' practices got better. It had taken a few years, but Tom Frieden and Farzad Mostashari had figured out a way to get independent doctors—the ones who served the city's poor—to do a better job at saving lives. The software worked. And it was touching the lives of three million New Yorkers.

• • •

We kept nudging other food companies to sign on to our salt plan. The publicity was all good, we told them. If giants like Kraft and Unilever could do it, so could they. The other food companies didn't rush, but by the fall of 2010 we had enough latecomers for a second announcement. Butterball promised to cut salt in its deli meats and hot dogs, Snyder's of Hanover to change its pretzels and chips, Heinz to move past ketchup to frozen pizza, and Hostess to cut sodium in its Wonder bread, snack cakes, and doughnuts. Then the supermarket group Delhaize America, which had sixteen hundred stores under names like Food Lion and Hannaford, promised that it would reduce the salt in its private-label products in twenty-two categories, including frozen pizza, cereal, and butter.

Many others still sat it out. But our conversations with two food companies showed that we were at least getting their attention. The first had come to us when we ran an ad campaign.

Whenever we talked to food companies, they complained that by adding salt, they were only meeting their customers' tastes. If we wanted them to use less salt, the corporations told us, we must educate consumers. I was irked that companies spending millions in advertising to persuade people to eat their unhealthy food then blamed their customers for being ignorant enough to eat it. But it was true that most people didn't know that too much salt was bad for them. In the fall of 2010 we put out ads to educate consumers. They weren't what the food companies had in mind.

The U.K.'s Food Standards Agency had run a three-stage education campaign. The first round told viewers that too much salt was bad, the second that people should eat less than 6 grams of salt (about 2,300 mg sodium) per day, and the third that packaged food was "full of it." They hoped to persuade people to compare labels and choose foods with less sodium. But we had no budget for salt advertising. Lynn Silver decided that if she could gather enough money for only one campaign, our message should be the FSA's third. We produced two ads, one featuring a can of soup and another a frozen dinner, each bursting with a snowstorm of salt. "Many foods pack a lot more salt than you think," the ads read. "TOO MUCH SALT CAN LEAD TO HEART ATTACK AND STROKE. Compare Labels. Choose Less Sodium."

The soup ad stirred up Denise Morrison, the incoming CEO of Campbell Soup. The ad, she complained, "suggests that salt is all that a consumer gets in a typical can of prepared soup. This is plainly untrue, and New Yorkers would not be well served by a campaign that persuades them to eat less soup."

Soon afterward, at Morrison's request, Andy Goodman, Sonia Angell, Lynn Silver, Christine Curtis, Kelly Christ, and I sat at the conference table in my office with Campbell's CEO and four of her senior staff for a soup tasting. Campbell, the executives told us, sold more than 60 percent of the canned soup in America and had been working to reduce sodium in its soup for decades. In recent years it had cut the sodium by a third in its tomato soup, which they said fed 25 million households in America. Campbell had also started a line of low-sodium soups called Healthy Request.

If they hoped to show us that Campbell had made progress, they succeeded. Their tomato soup already had less sodium than the targets we had set for 2014, and I thought it was tasty. With Campbell's tomato soup such a staple of the American diet, that achievement was helping prevent high blood pressure across the country. But if the executives hoped to prove that Campbell couldn't do more, they failed. The Healthy Request line of low sodium soups made up only 10 percent of its sales, which confirmed what all the food companies know: labeling a food "low sodium" drives down sales because customers assume it tastes bad. Most of Campbell's red-and-white canned soups—other than tomato—in my grocery store had nearly 900 mg of sodium per one-cup serving. That was more than our target and more than half of the sodium that most people should eat in an entire day. (Sylvia Birnbaum's favorite, Butternut Squash Bisque, had a little less salt than that but still more than our target for 2012.) So Campbell had shown that it could cut the salt in mainstream soups and win with customers. It just needed to do that for more types. Later, Campbell joined the NSRI but only for its canned food (SpaghettiOs) line.

A certain giant of the food industry, one that most people didn't think of as a food company, had been ignoring us. Walmart was now a major grocery store. By 2010 it was selling between 15 and 20 percent of the groceries in America. In January 2011 its executives appeared in the national news, beside Michelle Obama, promising to "make food healthier." By coincidence, around the same time Walmart was trying get Mayor Bloomberg's support, over fierce union resistance, to open stores in New York City. Trying to show a friendly face, it sent Andrea Thomas, its senior vice president for sustainability, to meet with me and other city officials in City Hall.

Thomas's Healthier Food plan sounded serious. By 2015, she said, Walmart would eliminate all artificial trans fats, cut added sugars by 10 percent in dairy items, sauces, and fruit drinks, and cut sodium by 25 percent in many categories of foods. The salt reduction requirement covered breads, meats, cheese, sauces, condiments, snacks, and packaged prepared foods. She would apply it to both private-label and branded products. Walmart's market share was so big, I figured, that every major food manufacturer in America would have to meet its demands. Unlike the FDA, which was obligated to spend years parrying industry protests before issuing rules, Walmart could rule by decree.

This one woman, I thought, had more power over the food industry than that massive government food agency in Washington. It was a lesson as much in the feebleness of our public health agencies as in the market dominance of Walmart. I left the meeting skeptical about how the company would enforce her plan or even measure progress. The industry introduced and discontinued thousands of products every year, and

Walmart didn't have someone like Christine Curtis calculating sales-weighted average sodium levels from databases. Still, my head was spinning about the potential impact. I was most shocked, though, when I asked Thomas why she had decided to reduce salt by 25 percent. We got that from you, she said.

. . .

The federal government's attitude was painfully different. After the toothless HHS Nutrition Summit and the disappearing act by the federal health agencies, I decided to press a little. The food companies kept telling us that because they distributed their food nationally, the government for the whole nation should be in charge. They had a point. In a better world, the FDA would drive the initiative, with the other health agencies cheering them on.

In June 2011 I wrote to HHS secretary Kathleen Sebelius, urging her to "make sodium reduction a national public health priority" based on the Institute of Medicine report. I also asked for a meeting with Sam Kass, the personal chef and close friend to the Obamas who was running Michelle Obama's Let's Move! childhood obesity initiative. He now had the title of Senior Policy Adviser for Nutrition in the White House.

Kass was a muscular former college baseball player with a shaved head and a gruff manner. He didn't respond much to my ideas on trans fats or nutrition standards for government-purchased foods, but he got animated when I brought up salt. The problem, he said, raising his voice, is "no one ever thinks about taste. *No one* thinks about *taste!*"

I don't know what kind of pressure the food companies or members of Congress might have put on him. Still, I was dumbfounded. Did he really think that we had worked on this for years without considering humans' taste for salt?

And then I wondered if I weren't looking at the roadblock. Was a man in the White House trained as a chef telling Tom Frieden and FDA commissioner Margaret Hamburg that they couldn't utter a word on salt? It was an unsettling thought.

14

"We are in a coalition with
major food companies for
one reason only; that is,
access to power."

The death of the soda tax in the spring of 2010 had been painful to watch. Every single year the obesity epidemic was killing far more Americans than were killed in the entire Vietnam War. The tax died not because it wouldn't slow the epidemic or because the issue was complicated; the soda companies killed it. The soda industry was infiltrated everywhere—with bottling plants dotted across the state, restaurants and convenience stores in every neighborhood, and vending machines even in schools. All of them got a piece of the business and resisted any attempt to change it. The American Beverage Association didn't have the street-fighter image of the NRA or the sinister reputation of the tobacco companies, but to me it looked more powerful.

The soda companies' arguments against the tax were hollow. But if any had struck a chord with New Yorkers, it was that the government was just using the obesity epidemic to squeeze people for their money. And that made me think of a different angle.

In June 2010, Robert Doar, the commissioner of the city's main social service agency, and I drove to Albany to meet with the commissioner of the state's Office of Temporary and Disability Assistance (OTDA). We brought ideas about the Supplemental Nutrition Assistance Program (SNAP), which pays for groceries for low-income people. It was once called Food Stamps.

President Franklin Roosevelt had created Food Stamps during the depths of Great Depression to protect farmers from being crushed by collapsing food prices. At that time, Americans had to buy the stamps, some of which they could redeem only for farm commodities. The Department of Agriculture, which ran the program, ended it as the economy strengthened in World War II, but Lyndon Johnson revived it with his War on Poverty. In the late 1970s the federal government started giving out the stamps for free instead of selling them.

The program had grown since then, keeping its political support even when the entire nation turned against welfare programs, because it was about food. Even staunch conservatives didn't think poor people should starve in America. In the early 2000s the USDA replaced the stamps with electronic benefit transfer (EBT) cards. In 2008 it rebranded Food Stamps as "supplemental nutrition assistance" to emphasize that the program, rather than holding back starvation, helped people get healthy food. In 2008 the USDA was running a $30 million demonstration project in which participants got extra value to their benefits if they used them to buy fruits and vegetables. During the recession that followed the mortgage security crash, SNAP grew to new heights. By 2013 the enormous program reached 48 million people, or 14 percent of Americans, and paid for $76 billion in food a year.

Across the nation, SNAP funds bought mountains of unhealthy food, like candy, chips, snack cakes, and soda. In 2010, about $5 billion a year from SNAP paid just for sugary drinks. That was five times CDC's budget to prevent chronic diseases.

I thought the SNAP rules should match its new name and actually assist with nutrition. Only Congress could change the rules permanently, but the USDA could authorize limited demonstration projects.

Any request to the USDA for a demonstration project, though, could be made only by state agencies that managed SNAP, which in New York was OTDA.

In Albany, Doar and I suggested three ideas to the OTDA commissioner. We could set health standards for foods that were eligible under SNAP. We could give SNAP recipients extra benefits to buy fruits and vegetables. Or we could require grocery stores participating in the program to stock or promote healthier items. The commissioner warmed to the ideas but thought most were too complicated for her agency to manage under complicated federal rules. In the end, we settled on the simplest change.

In October 2010, Mayor Bloomberg and Governor Paterson announced that New York State was submitting a request to the USDA for a two-year demonstration project that would remove sugary drinks from the SNAP program. It hadn't taken much to get the governor and the mayor behind the idea. State health commissioner Richard Daines and I argued that the government shouldn't buy, and then hand out for free, the food that was the single biggest contributor to our nation's number-one nutritional problem—at all, but especially in the name of a nutrition program. The rule change wouldn't affect the size of the benefit; SNAP participants would get every penny of their monthly food allowance.

This idea wasn't new or radical. When Congress revived Food Stamps in 1964, the House version of the bill had excluded soda. Aside from SNAP, no federal nutrition program in 2008 included sugary drinks. The school lunch program certainly didn't allow them. The Special Supplemental Nutrition Program for Women, Infants, and Children—known as WIC—gave mothers vouchers for only a short list of food items, and soda wasn't one. Interestingly, in 2009, when the USDA strengthened the nutrition criteria for the WIC "food package," children on WIC began eating healthier food, and stores began stocking healthier items. If WIC could change both Americans' diets and what was on grocery shelves, so could SNAP.

It wouldn't have been a big change to the program. SNAP benefits are not cash. You can't use them to buy cigarettes or beer. You can't use them to buy pet food, paper towels, vitamins, or chewing gum, none of which the USDA considers food. And you can't use them to buy meals in restaurants or even deli sandwiches in grocery stores. Our proposal would just add one more item to the excluded list.

And it wouldn't have been a big change for people enrolled in SNAP. For most people, the average SNAP benefit of $133 per person each month was too little to cover the entire grocery bill. SNAP is a supplement. Families enrolled in SNAP used their own money after their monthly benefits ran out and to buy excluded items. If SNAP participants wanted to buy soda (instead of drinking water for free), they could spend their own money for it. And then they could use the SNAP benefits not spent on soda to purchase healthier foods.

Because we were proposing a demonstration project, we had to evaluate it. To write the evaluation plan, I turned to a young health department doctor, Susan Kansagra.

Kansagra has short brown hair and is petite, unassuming, and quick to laugh. She is also, I learned, confident in herself and brainy even among the health department's whiz kids. She grew up in Greenville, South Carolina, the daughter of a pharmacist who immigrated from India. Like Amanda Parsons, in college she had considered a career in business. Then one day, while flipping through a magazine in her ophthalmologist's waiting room, Kansagra saw a photo of a woman with a stethoscope around her neck, holding an African baby. That picture somehow struck a chord. She quietly tore out the picture, took it home, and headed to medical school.

In 2008, after finishing her residency at Harvard, Kansagra looked for jobs in New York. Also like Parsons, she heard that exciting things were happening at the health department, so she managed to get her CV into Tom Frieden's e-mail inbox. He hired her to find and synthesize scientific evidence for him. In the first six months, she read so many scientific papers that she had to buy reading glasses because of the eyestrain. When I replaced Frieden, I asked her to help with the department's drawn-out response to H1N1 influenza, then increasingly relied on her for initiatives to prevent chronic diseases.

We didn't want to give the USDA excuses to reject our SNAP proposal, so Kansagra's evaluation plan for it was scientifically rigorous. She would repeatedly survey 4,200 SNAP participants in New York City and—as a comparison—in neighboring counties, asking about purchases and consumption of sugary drinks. She would also get data on sales of sugary drinks from grocery stores, before and after the policy change. She didn't know how many people the rule change would prompt to buy less soda, but even a 20 percent drop in sugary drink consumption would help slow obesity, and her study could detect a drop much smaller than that. Because the USDA cared very much about SNAP users' feeling ashamed to use their benefits, she proposed to include questions on stigma in the surveys.

The SNAP proposal stirred up the press, roused opinion writers, and scrambled the usual political lineup. Most people viewed our other ideas as liberal, but Republicans and conservatives tended to like the SNAP proposal, and Democrats and liberals generally didn't. At the same time Bill de Blasio, a staunch liberal who was then the city's public advocate, endorsed it.

But the proposal enraged the soda companies. The day after our announcement, Coca-Cola CEO Muhtar Kent sent a letter to Bloomberg, calling the idea "unjustified and discriminatory." PepsiCo CEO Indra Nooyi, writing the same day, was more threatening. "When we met earlier this summer," she told the mayor, "we let you know that as we restructure our business, we are redoubling our commitment to retain and increase our investment in New York City and New York State. But apparently commitment and loyalty is a one-way street in New York. Since our meeting, attacks on our business by the City of New York have gone unabated. . . . I am particularly concerned that you have chose [sic] to focus on just one category, and assault it across the board. I am sincerely hoping we can meet and talk about how we can work together."

I don't know what the soda companies were saying to the USDA, but I doubt it was gentle. Days later the grocery stores complained to the agency: the Food Industry Alliance of New York State wrote that "no food inherently is bad within the context of a balanced diet. . . . Yet, by government imposing its directive into food choices . . . SNAP shoppers will be deprived of nutritional decisions heretofore left to their discretion." It would be too complicated to distinguish sugary drinks from low- and no-calorie drinks, the stores wrote, because "with new product introductions or a change in formulary, computer checkouts need to be re-programmed, cashiers need to be educated, etc." And knowing that the USDA cared deeply about the stigma of using SNAP, the stores claimed that "not only will SNAP shoppers feel different, they will also be treated differently than other customers." The stores also argued that people might travel to the suburbs just to buy soda with SNAP.

All their arguments were bogus. To say that "no food inherently is bad within the context of a balanced diet" is to say that no food on grocery shelves is so toxic that it kills you quickly. That's a low bar for deciding what to include in a nutrition assistance program. Grocery stores already had to regularly reprogram their checkout computers to distinguish items like chewing gum that were not SNAP eligible from items like candy that were; reprogramming them to distinguish Coke from Diet Coke couldn't be difficult. As for SNAP shoppers, at checkout they already swiped an EBT card for their SNAP-eligible items, then swiped a credit or debit card or paid cash for everything else; nothing in our rule would change that, so it was hard to see how it would increase stigma. Finally, the idea that people would drive across the George Washington Bridge, paying a toll of at least $8, to buy soda with an EBT card was laughable.

The public face of the opposition, though, was not the soda companies or the grocery stores. It was "antihunger" organizations that ran food banks and advocated for SNAP. The same day the grocery store letter hit the USDA, the widely quoted antihunger activist Joel Berg sent the agency his own fiery eight-page letter. Under screaming heads like "THE PROPOSAL WOULD PUNISH LOW-INCOME PEOPLE FOR THE SUPPOSED CRIME OF BEING POOR," he wrote that our proposal "violates the law, restricts freedom, and criminalizes hunger by eliminating the ability of low-income SNAP recipients to even occasionally obtain sugar-sweetened beverages."

The antihunger activists were cozy with the big food companies. Feeding America, a national network of two hundred food banks, has a board with members from ConAgra, General Mills, Mars, Kroger, Walmart, and Nationwide Agribusiness. And they looked well connected to the soda companies too; the spokesman for the American Beverage Association told the *Times*, "Fighting hunger is a pretty heavy lift. I think we need all the hands we can get working on that cause. I don't see a conflict here." The antihunger groups didn't seem ashamed about doing the bidding of the big food corporations. Edward Cooney, executive director of the Congressional Hunger Center, told the *Times*, "We are in a coalition with major food companies for one reason only; that is, access to power."

• • •

In the summer of 2010, when we compiled the results of the previous year's telephone surveys, we perked up. Beginning in 2007, we had included questions on sugary drinks on the surveys, and over the next two years the percent of New Yorkers who said they drank one or more a day dropped from 36 to 32 percent. That translated to a fall of more than 250,000 New Yorkers. Was it possible that the media attention given to sugary drinks—not just our ads but also the fights over soda taxes—was persuading people to avoid soda?

We weren't sure, but we decided to keep making noise. The early focus groups on sugary drinks had given advertising man Jose Bandujo another idea. "What are these *grams* that are on these cans and bottles?" he said. "Nobody knows what a gram of sugar is." He decided to translate it into something people understood. When he did, his team was shocked.

They came up with two subway posters. One showed a 20-ounce bottle of soda, with the headline "YOU JUST ATE 16 PACKS OF SUGAR." The other pictured a 32-ounce cup, with the words "YOUR KID JUST ATE 26 PACKS OF SUGAR." In both, sugar packs poured into the containers, which then overflowed with blubber.

That same summer employees of both Coke and Pepsi asked to meet with us. They wanted to tell us about work they were planning in the Bronx. It was New York City's poorest borough and the county that routinely ranked last in the state in nearly every health statistic. People in the Bronx drank the most soda and were the most overweight.

The two soda companies' campaigns were close cousins. Pepsi's "Zero Calorie Bronx Test" meant pushing its diet brands, such as its new Pepsi Max, by putting more bottles on store shelves, installing special in-store display racks, distributing discount coupons, and running street "sampling" events with a truck labeled "Fantastico Sabor. No Incluye Calorias." Coke's "Bronx Pilot" tried to increase sales of its diet drink, especially Coke Zero, with billboards, in-store display racks and ads, meal tie-ins, coupons, bundles ("Buy three 2-liter bottles and get one 2-liter bottle free"), and a sampling truck emblazoned with "Real Coca-Cola Taste and Zero Calories." Both companies also touted money they were giving to community groups: Pepsi was funding four churches to teach people to eat fruits and vegetables, and Coke was giving grants to schools for exercise programs that reached a few hundred children.

Both companies were master marketers, brilliant at driving sales of their products. But their marketing in the Bronx would just pump up sales of their diet brands, not cut sales of their full-sugar brands. The rest was politics and public relations. Reaching a few hundred kids in the Bronx would buy them some valuable friends in the most stricken neighborhoods and make for good talking points for lobbyists, but it wasn't going to touch the obesity epidemic in a borough of 1.4 million.

I couldn't help but wonder if their plans were connected to something else that had happened that summer. Lawyer David Grandeau had recently filed a request under the state's Freedom of Information Law (FOIL) about our *Pouring on the Pounds* campaign. He was following the money, asking for invoices, payments, and the names of donors who had helped pay for the counter-ads. When I asked him later for whom he was making the request, he refused to tell me. The state's FOIL law doesn't require the agency to release documents that are "deliberative," which meant nearly all our e-mails were protected. But because of an internal screw-up, our agency sent Grandeau a pack of e-mails anyway. He forwarded them to his client, who must have tipped off *Times* reporter Anemona Harticollis, because we soon got a FOIL request from her that was an exact duplicate of his. Our office sent her the same packet.

The e-mails bared the back-and-forth behind the statement in the video that "drinking 1 can of soda a day . . . can make you 10 pounds fatter a year." The messages were far too juicy for any reporter to resist. "Behind this simple claim," Harticollis wrote in the *Times*, "was a protracted dispute in the department over the scientific validity of directly linking sugar consumption to weight gain—one in which the city's health commissioner, Dr. Thomas A. Farley, overruled three subordinates, including his chief nutritionist." She quoted health department dietitian Cathy Nonas writing that, "As we get into this exacting science, the idea of a sugary drink becoming fat is absurd." Scientists, she wrote, "will make mincemeat of us." Harticollis quoted scientific experts confirming that drinking sugary drinks tended to add fat but adding that how much depended on exercise and overall calorie consumption. And in one of the e-mails, a Columbia University obesity expert Michael Rosenbaum wrote, "Basic premise doesn't work."

As we had haggled and consulted experts over powerful wording that we could stand behind, Cathy Nonas had used a very unfortunate phrase: "What can we get away with?" Harticollis wrote that the e-mails "show what happens when officials try to balance science and public relations and toe the line between disseminating information and lobbying for a cause."

Other newspapers weren't as forgiving. The *Post*'s headline was "SUGARY AD A BIG FAT 'LIE.'" The paper's editorial the next day said "Farley's claim to credibility—to legitimacy—is that he is a scientist, a man whose principal allegiance is to the truth. But it turns out that he is just another administration propagandist. . . . Tom Farley lied. That should matter."

For the record, the body does convert sugar into fat in part, and the insulin surge provoked by drinking sugary drinks causes the body to store fat. The idea that consuming sugar makes you fat was the key argument that scientists were making to explain the obesity epidemic. I can defend the ten-pound number, too: when researchers "overfed" volunteers 1,000 calories a day, six days a week, for fourteen weeks, the people gained between 9 and 29 pounds, a rate that translates to between 6 and 19 pounds from "overfeeding" one can of soda per day for a year. And "overfeeding" sugary drinks is exactly what happens in the real world, because sugary drinks tend to be added to the diet rather than replacing food.

We put out a press statement that we stood by our ten-pound claim. It was the result of "vigorous internal discussion" that "is part of any scientifically sound decision-making process, but usually occurs outside of public view." Dr. Rosenbaum wrote a letter to the *Times* backing us up. Still, I should have put a disclaimer in the ad saying that the number assumed no other changes in diet or physical activity. I was sloppy with the wording, and my credibility took a hit.

The bigger lesson I learned, though, was that the soda companies were no longer willing to just play defense.

• • •

Although the USDA could rule on the SNAP demonstration project on its own, it listens to Congress. And Congress listens to lobbyists. I heard from New York City's Washington office that as soon as we announced our idea, the American Beverage Association was lobbying black and Hispanic members against it. So within two weeks of our announcement I went to Washington to present our side.

The congressional staffers most familiar with SNAP gave me the weary responses of those who had been fighting to a stalemate for too long. The idea of restricting SNAP to healthy foods had come up before, they said, but it never made any headway. Republicans generally weren't enthusiastic about SNAP, and many wanted to cut funding for it; fiddling with the rules didn't excite them. Democrats saw a split in their advocacy groups: some health organizations pushed for nutrition criteria while the antihunger groups fiercely fought them; the fact that the antihunger groups were in bed with the big food companies didn't seem to matter. With the opposition fragmented, the big food companies had free rein, so junk food and beverages stayed in the nutrition program.

Another two weeks later, Robert Doar, New York State health commissioner Richard Daines, and I went to the USDA's headquarters in Washington, a building that fills a giant city block along the Mall. We met with Under Secretary Kevin Concannon, who oversaw all of the USDA's food programs. Concannon, a white-haired former social worker with a genial manner and a Maine accent, had nearly a dozen of his staff with him.

I made the health argument with dense slides showing facts, numbers, and graphs, and explained how scientifically rigorous our evaluation plan was. Doar talked about the growth of the SNAP program in New York City (more recipients being better in the eyes of the USDA) and how our proposed change wasn't administratively difficult. But it was Daines—a Mormon with conservative politics—who made the most powerful argument. He spoke of walking across the boundary from the Upper East Side to Harlem and being incensed by the sudden onslaught of bodegas hawking sugary drinks. It just wasn't right, he said, to help the beverage companies profit by getting poor black kids fat on soda.

Concannon looked genuinely interested, asking a few questions and joking that he had a support group within the USDA called Change Has a Small Constituency. But some of his deputies sounded hostile to the idea. One even suggested that restricting sugary drinks might make them a status symbol in poor neighborhoods and actually increase sales. Concannon called our proposal "a momentous experiment," on a scale that the USDA had never done before. If it happened, an evaluation would be crucial to "isolate" the effect of the sugary drink prohibition from other changes.

. . .

I kept pressing my staff for more ideas on obesity. From my early days in the health department, Lynn Silver kept coming back to the problem of ballooning portion sizes—a problem that she felt carried its own solution.

In the early 2000s, researchers were churning out studies highlighting an unnerving fact of human nature: when people are served bigger portions, they just eat more. Nutrition researcher Barbara Rolls had invited 51 men and women into her laboratory for lunch on four different days, offering them different portions of Kraft macaroni and cheese. Even the smallest portion—about 7 cups—was huge. When she served her volunteers a portion twice as large as that, they ate 160 more calories than when she served them the smaller portion, without feeling any more full. "Most people are unaware of what constitutes an appropriate portion size," Dr. Rolls wrote. "Thus, the ready availability of foods in large portions is likely to be facilitating the overconsumption of energy in many persons."

She found the same unsettling portion-size effect with deli sandwiches, bags of potato chips, fruits and vegetables, and soda. People served 18-ounce glasses of Pepsi at lunch drank more than when they were served 12-ounce glasses. The behavior lasted, too. In one study, people given 50 percent larger portions at every meal ate and drank more for eleven straight days. They took in an astonishing 420 extra calories a day, or more than enough to gain an extra pound in just that week and a half.

In the most devious study, researcher Brian Wansink at Cornell invented soup bowls that he could secretly refill from the bottom as people ate. When he offered study volunteers a meal of tomato soup, those eating from the refilling bowls ate 73 percent more soup than those who ate from regular bowls. And like almost all the people in these studies, they were oblivious that they had consumed more. For all our vanity about our ability to reason, we humans often behave like passive receptacles for whatever food is within arm's reach.

Restaurants didn't publish studies like these, but the cancerous growth of portion sizes showed that they understood the principle. When McDonald's opened in the 1950s, it offered only one size order of French fries: 2.4 ounces. By 1999, it sold a "large" that was two and a half times that, and a "Super Size" that was three times that. And that was nothing compared to soda. In the 1950s, the only size cup on the menu was 7 ounces. In 2003 two of the choices were a 32-ounce "large" and a 42-ounce "Super Size"—six times the 1950s portion. After 2004's stinging *Super Size Me* documentary, McDonald's shrank its cup sizes somewhat, but in 2010 a "medium" drink at McDonald's was 21 ounces—three times the only size in the 1950s. And McDonald's was responsible compared to KFC, which sold sodas in half-gallon tubs delivering 54 packets of sugar. Restaurants come out ahead with even small price increases for their bigger sizes, so they set prices that nudge people to larger ones. At Checkers in New York City, a 12-ounce "Kids"-size drink cost 9.1 cents per ounce, but a 42-ounce "large" cost only 5.0 cents per ounce.

In theory, the solution is simple: give people food in portions appropriate to human needs. Even if they can choose seconds, they usually won't. In Barbara Rolls's studies, people who were given smaller portions ate less but were just as satisfied. In the 1950s, people weren't dissatisfied with their portion sizes. And they were thinner.

Lynn Silver thought the only way to restore human-size portions was to require them. Restaurants wouldn't do it voluntarily, no matter how much we might ask or cajole them; their profits depended too much on the big sizes. The easiest item for which to set a maximum size was a drink, because the portion matched the size of the container. There was no such simple way to judge the size of a burger or a pile of fries. The portion cap for sugary drinks met her Holy Grail criteria—low cost, high impact, big reach—and it had the extra advantage that it avoided "the whole political dimension of taxes."

The idea of capping portion sizes to fight obesity was new. When Silver first proposed it, I thought it was brilliant—and I dismissed it. I had no doubt that if we could enact the rule, people would drink less. But the appearance and the politics of it stopped me dead. Even though portion sizes were determined not by customers but by restaurants, the customers had the illusion that what they ate was their choice alone. The public and the politicians would reject a portion cap as an interference with that choice.

I asked Silver instead to come up with a plan to restore human-size portions in restaurants, one that included not just sugary drinks but also French fries and sandwiches, and that was voluntary. There must be some way we could give a health department seal of approval—or even a financial bonus—to restaurants that served food in sizes that didn't get their customers fat. She felt certain that too few restaurants would care about any incentive for the program to work. I told her to try anyway.

She came back with lists of ideas, none of which looked promising. Her staff investigated "healthy restaurant" programs elsewhere. None of them was working, because the only restaurants with the time and interest to get the seal of approval were the chains, even if the criteria were lax. None of us wanted McDonald's—and only McDonald's—to

get a "healthy restaurant" stamp because it offered a couple of small sandwiches within a huge unhealthy menu.

I asked other staff members for ideas and e-mailed a few half-baked
suggestions of my own. We went back and forth for nearly a year and a
half. "We went through so many different iterations on what [a voluntary
plan] could possibly be," recalled Maura Kennelly. Lynn Silver became
deeply frustrated that I kept demanding a voluntary scheme. "We just
kept hitting a wall," said another staff person who worked on it. Nothing
seemed legal, practical, and effective.

We were all exasperated. Finally, in the summer of 2011, I asked Andy
Goodman and Lynn Silver to show me in detail how we might design a
portion cap for sugary drinks that was mandatory.

. . .

In April 2011 eighteen members of the Congressional Black Caucus,
including the ranking Democratic member of the House subcommittee
overseeing the USDA, sent a letter to USDA secretary Thomas Vilsack
attacking our proposal to restrict SNAP purchases of sugary drinks. Their
words sounded much like those of the food companies. The proposal
would "unfairly treat SNAP customers differently from other customers,
unduly complicate SNAP redemption at the point of sale and threaten to
increase the stigma long associated with SNAP."

Four months later, and ten months after we submitted our proposal,
the USDA turned us down. The "scale and scope" were too large and
complex, the department wrote; there were "a number of unresolved
operational challenges and complexities," and "the proposed evaluation
design is not adequate."

The department would consider, though, "potential alternative col-
laborations such as a public-private partnership to design, implement, and
evaluate an anti-obesity intervention targeting consumption and associated behaviors while encouraging healthy choices." And staffers hinted in
conversations afterward that they might approve a much smaller demonstration project in Staten Island, in which we combined the sugary drink

restriction with a "positive" incentive, like giving people extra SNAP benefits to buy vegetables.

Why Staten Island? I assumed it was because the complaints had come from the Congressional Black Caucus, and most people on Staten Island were white. Why combine the restriction with a "positive" incentive? Because people inside the USDA or in Congress viewed excluding sugary drinks—even though they were dangerous—as "negative." Why a "public-private partnership"? I could only guess that that meant the USDA would agree only if food companies or grocery stores didn't object.

I didn't like the idea of running the demonstration project in Staten Island when our highest obesity rates were in the Bronx. I didn't want to do a small research study when my job was to end an epidemic that was killing people citywide. And I wasn't enthusiastic about combining the restriction with a "positive" financial incentive, because that would definitely have made the evaluation design "not adequate."

But my biggest problem with the USDA's hinted-at invitation was that it wasn't ours to accept or not. The department dealt only with the State of New York, which since January 2011 had a new governor, Andrew Cuomo. And Cuomo had presidential ambitions. He barely spoke to his health commissioner, but he did send a clear message that he wouldn't do a thing on sugary drinks. We tried for many months to get the state under Cuomo to talk to the USDA about a revised proposal, but we got nowhere. And with that, our idea of changing SNAP rules to slow the obesity epidemic met the same death as the soda tax.

15

"They always had two nuclear weapons."

In late December 2010, federal court judge Jed Rakoff killed our rule requiring warning signs in stores selling cigarettes. He opened his opinion with a rhetorical flourish: "Even merchants of morbidity are entitled to the full protection of the law, for our sake as well as theirs." Federal law preempted our rule, he wrote, because the law prohibited states from enacting requirements "with respect to the advertising or promotion" of cigarettes. Rakoff decreed that the racks of cigarette packs qualified as "promotion" and that a rule requiring warning signs near the racks or the cash register "imposes burdens on the promotion of cigarettes that only the federal government may prescribe."

The health department's lawyer, Tom Merrill, believed that the tobacco industry accepted the federal cigarette laws only "because they always had two nuclear weapons. They had preemption, and they had the First Amendment." This time the tobacco companies had had to detonate only their first nuke.

When Anne Pearson, who had come up with the warning sign idea, got enough past her grieving to read the ruling, she couldn't fathom it. The federal law was about labeling of cigarette packs and advertising. The warning signs didn't touch either one. It had never occurred to her that a judge would declare cigarette packs themselves to be "promotion." Or that a judge would see a warning sign in the vicinity as somehow interfering with that promotion. "It really struck us as being apples and oranges," she said. The federal law was never "intended to tie of hands of a jurisdiction that wanted to give information to its citizens. Even with our rule in place, the retailers are absolutely free to promote their products." Under Rakoff's yawning interpretation, the federal law might block just about anything we would do to protect people from cigarette marketing, because it would impose a "burden on promotion." Pearson was devastated. "This proposal felt so much like one of my children, my baby," she told me years later. "It's still pretty painful."

The ruling was especially agonizing because the warning signs had been working. Before and after the signs went up in stores selling cigarettes, we had surveyed a thousand smokers and recent quitters as they exited. The surveys showed big increases in the percent who noticed a sign (from 30 to 67 percent), and among people who saw a sign, the percent whom the sign prompted to think about quitting "a lot" (from 34 to 47 percent).

Judge Rakoff wrote of high democratic principle. But I could only see the greater principle of the power of money in our democracy. The tobacco companies had persuaded a U.S. Congress hungry for campaign donations to pass laws prohibiting state and local governments from protecting their citizens from tobacco marketing. Then those same companies hired armies of brilliant lawyers to enforce the broadest possible interpretations of those prohibitions in court. Street-corner heroin dealers were also "merchants of morbidity," whose product killed far fewer people than were killed by tobacco, but they didn't get the "full protection of the law" that tobacco dealers did. The difference was not a democratic principle but rather simply that the heroin dealers hadn't reinvested their profits in election campaigns and lobbyists to rewrite laws in their favor.

I had seen the warning signs as opening up retail stores as a new front in the war against R.J. Reynolds. We had lost the first battle. It wouldn't be the last.

. . .

The health department's media man Jeffrey Escoffier remembers calling advertiser Jose Bandujo about a problem. Escoffier had scheduled focus groups for the next week to test out some ideas for antismoking ads. Bandujo had been working on a concept that intrigued Escoffier, but the idea was still just words on a page. Escoffier needed something graphic—very graphic—to show this idea to the focus groups. He needed storyboards right away.

After seeing New Yorkers' powerful response to Ronaldo and Marie, Escoffier and Beth Kilgore wanted to run a campaign centered specifically on how smoking-induced illness made people suffer. When Bandujo heard about it, he was convinced they were on the right track. When other ads told people that smoking kills, smokers reacted by saying, as he put it, "I could get hit by a cab. Or an air conditioner is gonna fall on my head. I'm going to die anyway." Bandujo thought, "We gotta counteract that 'die anyway.'" As a child he had heard his uncle, who was dying of lung cancer, awakening day after day with coughing fits. "No one's talking about those ten years *before* you die," Bandujo said. One of his staff knew someone who had been incapacitated from a stroke. "You read the obituary . . . 'Died of a stroke.' Well, she was paralyzed in her bed for four years before her stroke actually killed her. " The suffering was so bad that, at the end, "death is a relief. Death is the easy part!"

Bandujo felt he couldn't communicate that idea with a storyboard. So he called a video producer, who gathered a few actors he knew, and the group spent a weekend in a friend's apartment. One actor played the part of a woman lying in bed incapacitated, another her husband. They used a handheld camera. "So this is your life," Bandujo said. "This is your husband changing your diaper because you had a stroke from smoking."

The ad Bandujo produced "was raw," said Bob Brothers, who worked on it with him. "It really felt like watching somebody as a voyeur."

What hurt most was the sound. There was no music and no voiceover. Just the sound of the woman's breathing—slow, labored, and painful. Jeffrey Escoffier called it "the horrible sound of someone dying." The ad's thirty seconds felt like forever.

Bandujo shot a second ad, too, this one in the kitchen. A man with an oxygen tube under his nose sits at a small table, very much alone. He is struggling to breathe, loudly. Then he begins coughing, more and more. He struggles even more to catch his breath as he coughs. That sound "would just send chills through your body," said Brothers. "You hear that cough, and you just cringe. It makes your hair stick up."

The health department staff found the ads wrenching. "Even for us, who had been seeing hard-hitting ads all along," said one, "we were like, that's *really* tough! . . . Even if you watched them two or three times— even the *fourth* time—they're still hard to watch."

Escoffier and Kilgore showed the ads to the focus groups. After each ad ended, there was just prolonged "stunned silence." It was awful for smokers to imagine, after a stroke, being helpless. And even more awful to imagine the indignity of having family members change their diapers. In one group, Bandujo remembers, the participants became so emotional that the moderator had to stop the conversation and give everyone a break. "I felt chills when I saw that," said one focus group participant. "It really made me want to quit smoking for good."

The stroke ad taught Escoffier and Kilgore something else about smokers. People who smoke can brush off thoughts of risk to themselves. But smokers are anguished to think that they might inflict suffering on their loved ones.

Christina Chang had to get approval from the City Hall communications staff, who routinely picked apart, and sometimes killed, ads that our team had crafted. They also found the ads painful to watch. But they objected to Bandujo's tagline, "Dying is the easy part." What would that do to viewers who were suicidal? The city should never say that dying is easy. Escoffier and Kilgore changed the wording. The final version reads "Dying from smoking is rarely quick . . . and never painless. When smoking leads to stroke, you can suffer every minute of every day."

The City Hall staff were still anxious that the ads were too disturbing. They insisted that Deputy Mayor Howard Wolfson watch them. Wolfson approved the coughing man but thought the stroke ad was too much. He demanded that the diaper changing be less explicit. The ad went back and forth between his team and Bandujo's. Wolfson kept asking for more changes to soften it, but afterward he still wasn't willing to let the ad air.

Christina Chang told me she was frustrated that New Yorkers might never see the stroke ad *because* it was so powerful. I commented that I bet Bloomberg would like it. That gave her an idea. The next time she spotted the mayor at his desk in the Bull Pen, she appeared at his side holding a laptop and ran the stroke ad for him. "That's great," he told her. "Go with it."

When the ads aired in March 2011, they hit viewers very hard. Beth Kilgore remembered, "We got *so* many complaints." The raw, lonely scenes of suffering were deeply upsetting. They made people so anxious that they couldn't sleep at night. Smokers didn't want their children to see the ads; the kids worried that their parents would end up like that. The stroke ad reminded people of caring for their own ailing parents. "That's terrible," said Kilgore, "but it really drove people to have a real emotional connection to it." And, she said, the ads provoked more calls to the Smokers' Quitline than any similar-size campaign.

Jose Bandujo said later, "For us, the greatest compliment is when our friends say, 'Oh my god! That is the most horrible ad! That is the worst ad ever! I can't stand listening to it . . . I have to turn the TV off.'"

. . .

When I got the smoking number from the telephone surveys collected in 2010, I called Mayor Bloomberg right away. His aides quickly scheduled a press conference. We announced the number in a big, sunlit room on the fourteenth floor of our glassy new headquarters building, with panoramic views of Queens through its floor-to-ceiling windows. Bloomberg stood behind his mayoral podium, flanked by several video screens, facing rows of seated reporters and the news video cameras beyond them. He was ebullient. It was his "I told you so" moment. The smoking rate was now 14.0 percent, down another 100,000 smokers from the year before. New York City now had 450,000 fewer smokers than it had when he was elected, after a decade in which the number hadn't budged.

"When we came into office, we decided that controlling smoking was the single most important thing we could do to make life in New York healthier," Bloomberg told the reporters. And he rattled off the policies and programs that had worked: "our trailblazing Smoke-Free Air Act," hard-hitting media campaigns, making smoking cessation programs more widely available, and cigarette taxes.

Michael Bloomberg—an engineer, bond trader, and techie—loved data. Even as mayor, he kept a Bloomberg Terminal on his desk, tracking the markets with numbers and colorful graphs. But the numbers he showed that morning were the best ever: pictures of how he was saving lives. He took the reporters through graphs, slide after slide. The smoking rate had fallen by 43 percent among young adults. It had fallen by 40 percent among blacks. It had fallen by 50 percent on Staten Island. Among teenagers it had dropped by more than half, to the lowest rate ever recorded.

A year earlier, when the smoking rate was 15.8 percent, I had wondered what effect that drop in smoking since 2002 would do for New Yorkers over the long term. I asked department epidemiologist Sharon Perlman to project how many deaths would be prevented by the decline in smoking since Tom Frieden began. She came back with an estimate: over the next fifty years, she told me, the fall would save 100,000 New Yorkers from smoking-caused deaths. Could it really that many? I asked. Then we realized that the number was high in part because the model gave us credit if we prevented smoking-caused lung cancer in an eighty-two-year-old, even if that person were bound to die at age eighty-three from unrelated causes. That didn't feel like a great achievement.

I asked Perlman to try again, but this time to only count a "smoking death prevented" if the cancer or heart disease death were to happen before age seventy-five, when most people still have several good years of life left. She came back saying the health department's actions would prevent 50,000 deaths—much lower but still enough to make me dizzy: an average of one thousand lives saved per year, even if smoking rates in New York

City didn't fall any further. Most of those deaths would be prevented years in the future, but some people were already living longer and healthier because of our efforts. At the press conference, Bloomberg showed a graph with Perlman's projections, pointing out the 50,000 New Yorkers who were to avoid "premature, and usually painful, smoking-related deaths."

And then he dropped another statistic on the reporters. Of all the thousands of numbers he reviewed as mayor, Bloomberg's favorite was life expectancy. He believed it measured everything his administration cared about, from crime fighting to fire prevention to cleaner air. He once said life expectancy was the only number he wanted on his tombstone. And life expectancy at birth in New York City was growing surprisingly fast: between 2001 and 2008, it increased by 2.3 years, from 77.9 to 80.2. New York was also fast outpacing the rest of the country—it had opened up a gap in life expectancy with the rest of the United States of 2.1 years, greater than any in history. We couldn't prove that the plummeting smoking rate contributed to New York's surging life expectancy, but it was the best explanation we had.

By then, news of New York City's antismoking work was rippling across the world. The global tobacco control program, now run by Kelly Henning at Bloomberg's foundation, reached deeply into the fifteen low-income countries with the most smokers and helped another sixty smaller countries. Poor nations in which tobacco companies had been aggressively marketing were now passing smoke-free air laws, raising cigarette taxes, and banning cigarette advertising, following Tom Frieden's MPOWER model and using Bloomberg's money. And the ads New York City had created traveled too. Focus groups nearly everywhere were shaken by *Cigarettes Are Eating You Alive*, the gruesome ad with close-ups of cancers of the lip and neck that the agency developed in 2006, and a related ad *Cigarettes Are Eating Your Baby Alive*, which emphasized the effect of secondhand smoke on children. By the end of 2011, one or the other ad had played in China, India, Russia, Ukraine, Poland, Mexico, the Philippines, Vietnam, and Indonesia. For Mayor Bloomberg in New York City that day, it was a moment of triumph over death and suffering, the likes of which few others could ever claim.

"I remember that everyone was so happy," said Christina Chang, who watched from the wings. "It was one of the few moments when everyone was buoyant and felt victorious." Even Stu Loeser, Bloomberg's brooding press secretary, was smiling.

But as the mayor reveled in the graphs and numbers, showing slide after slide, Chang looked out at the crowd of battle-hardened reporters and saw something different. She thought, "God, they are so bored."

. . .

In 2010, after Sarah Perl took a job in another part of the health department, I asked Susan Kansagra to run its antitobacco program. That meant it fell to her to try again in retail stores. With our court loss over the warning sign rule still a raw wound, she hired a lawyer to work within her office to push the agenda while avoiding future losses.

Kevin Schroth, a tall, broad-shouldered triathlete, speaks in slow, careful, lawyerly phrases. His first job after law school was in a firm that represented the tobacco giant Lorillard. His experience taught him the "immense power that these law firms have and how much money and resources they can throw at a problem." When his father, a long-term ex-smoker, died of tongue and esophageal cancer, Schroth began searching for a job on the other side. On his first day at the health department, Susan Kansagra asked him to review a pair of policy ideas that he would stay with for the next two and a half years.

On his first day, Schroth met Vicki Grimshaw, an intense but soft-spoken member of the antitobacco program. Grimshaw had been immersing herself in the world of tobacco products and the tobacco companies' marketing tricks. She and Schroth became the team—practical and legal—that drove the antitobacco program's policy agenda for the rest of Bloomberg's third term.

The tobacco control staff at the New York State health department had pressed on Grimshaw an idea for retail stores: to mount a direct attack on the power walls. Back when we were surveying smokers about the warning signs, we had asked those who bought cigarettes on impulse what had prompted their purchase. The three most common triggers were the sight of the packs themselves, the price promotions, and the ads, in that order. Another study showed how much the displays affected children. A group of researchers asked more than a thousand middle-school students who had never tried smoking to list the convenience stores they visited. The researchers then went to those stores to count the cigarette packs and ads. A year later, when the researchers surveyed the children again, they found that those who had seen the most cigarette packs and ads were more than twice as likely to have tried smoking as those who saw the least. That made the ads a more powerful influence on children's starting to smoke than having a parent who smoked.

In fighting the power walls, New York City and the rest of the country lagged behind. Iceland led the world in 2001 when it passed a law requiring stores to keep cigarette packs out of view. Stores there kept cigarettes hidden in plain cabinets or behind curtains. Several provinces in Canada followed with their own bans on displaying tobacco products; then the idea spread to Australia, Ireland, and the U.K. After Ontario passed its law, smoking among teens dropped by 30 percent in a year.

The frustrating question for Kevin Schroth was whether U.S. courts would decide that the display of cigarette packs was "speech" that was protected by Bill of Rights. The U.S. Supreme Court hadn't viewed advertising—or "commercial speech"—as protected by the First Amendment until 1976, but since then the court had kept throwing more into the definition of what was protected. In 2007, in a frightening decision, the court said that a Vermont law prohibiting pharmacies from selling data to drug manufacturers on doctors' prescriptions was an unconstitutional restriction on speech. If selling private information was protected speech, then what wasn't?

The New York State health department hired lawyer Micah Berman to analyze how the court would handle a ban on displays of cigarette packs (but not the ads next to them). Berman thought such a ban would withstand a court challenge if the government could show that it would "advance the government's interest" in preventing kids from smoking but was "no more extensive than necessary." Or as Kevin Schroth put it, "You have to show that it works, but doesn't work too well."

"I was always nervous about it," health department general counsel Tom Merrill said of the pack display ban. It could too easily get squashed in the courts. He thought New York City's success in the calorie-labeling case had overly whetted the appetite of public health people for big policy victories. After that the Robert Wood Johnson Foundation had started funding lawyers to come up with more public health policy ideas. Merrill thought Berman's optimistic opinion on the cigarette display ban was just "a Robert Wood Johnson deliverable."

It was that. But if the tobacco companies paid many millions for power walls, those power walls must be driving sales, and if they were driving sales, we wanted them to disappear. A tobacco display ban in New York City would look different from one in Iceland or Canada, though. In the United States, the courts would force us to allow point-of-sale advertising, even if they permitted a ban on displaying the packs themselves. But later a study appeared suggesting that it was the packs that mattered. Researchers invited 1,200 teenagers to an online virtual-reality experiment. They randomly assigned the teens to different digital convenience stores that displayed cigarette packs, ads, both, or neither, and then asked the teens to "purchase" four items. When the packs were hidden, the teens were only one-third as likely to try to buy cigarettes, regardless of whether the virtual store had cigarette ads.

I didn't know if we would win in court or not, but I wanted to try. If we passed the rule, we at least had a chance to get rid of the power walls. If we didn't try, we would just concede the loss.

In late 2011 I took the idea to Mayor Bloomberg, showing him pictures of a pack-filled power wall in New York City and the plain cabinets in Canada. The tobacco companies would sue us, I told him, and we might not win. He liked the idea anyway and approved it on the spot. Unlike the earlier ideas that he had turned down, this one wouldn't prohibit stores from selling cigarettes. He felt any inconvenience to stores was worth it to prevent kids from smoking.

The city's Law Department, though, wanted to wait. The city had appealed our loss on the warning sign rule, and the lawyers wanted to first see how the court of appeals would define cigarette "promotion."

One other marketing ploy that the tobacco companies used in retail stores was manipulating prices. The companies kept prices (and profits) high for fully addicted smokers, but then tempted those trying to quit with discounts. They had three kinds of discounts: coupons ("$2 off!"), value-added incentives ("Buy 2 Packs, Get 1 Free!"), and specials ("Only $9.59!"). By 2010, 80 percent of the $8 billion in promotions from the tobacco companies were discounts. Our team found that one-quarter of smokers in the city had used some kind of discount—averaging $1.25 off—the last time they bought a pack. A pack-a-day smoker using discounts like these every day would see them as "saving" him or her over $400 a year.

In 2010 a network of lawyers called the Tobacco Control Legal Consortium began talking about laws to ban tobacco price discounts, and Vicki Grimshaw listened. When Kevin Schroth arrived, the discount ban was still just a raw idea. The two of them worked it into a bill that banned all three kinds of discounts and also set a minimum price.

Meanwhile Grimshaw, who spent time browsing in bodegas, discovered that the tobacco companies were getting creative with other forms of tobacco. "I found them selling two-for-sixty-nine-cents cigars," she said. "That didn't seem like a good idea when 'loosie' cigarettes have been illegal for a dozen years." She and Schroth added to the bill two other ideas: a requirement that little cigars be sold in packs of at least four, and additional enforcement authority for the city to prevent stores from selling smuggled cigarettes.

By the time Schroth and Grimshaw had worked out the details of the bill with other city agencies and I had gotten the mayor's approval, it was the summer of 2012. Bloomberg had less than eighteen months left in his final term. The City Council speaker Christine Quinn was leading the race to be the next mayor, and I was worried that she would avoid controversial bills during the election year. Our opportunity was closing fast. These two bills would be our last big swing at smoking.

16

"I hear that your mayor wants to ban soda!"

I n late 2011, despite our painful losses on the soda tax and the SNAP proposal, we saw signs of hope. Our 2010 telephone surveys showed New Yorkers continuing to turn against sugary drinks, with daily consumption now down to 30 percent (from 36 percent in 2007). Surveys of high school students were likewise showing big drops in soda drinking. And then in the summer of 2011, we were stunned to see falls in obesity itself. The city's public school system had begun weighing and measuring children in 2006, and by 2011, the proportion of children in elementary school who were obese had edged down from 21.9 to 20.7 percent. That wasn't much of a fall, but coming after forty years of relentless rises in childhood obesity, it signaled a tidal shift. The younger the children, the faster the obesity rates were falling. We didn't have dietary surveys of children, so we couldn't explain the reversal, but something good was happening.

It was far too early to declare victory, though. New Yorkers were still gulping soda and wolfing down junk food, and rates of obesity and diabetes kept hitting new heights in adults. If we wanted to prevent thousands of New Yorkers from getting amputations or going on dialysis every year, we needed to press on. While we weren't forgetting junk food, we took the hint of progress as a reason to push harder on soda. And as we took a third big stab at sugary drinks, we introduced an idea that was heard around the world.

In November 2011, Lynn Silver, Susan Kansagra, Maura Kennelly, Christina Chang, and about ten others filled the seats around a long conference table next to my office in our new headquarters. They were there to explain how we could limit the portion size for sugary drinks in restaurants. It was an odd meeting, because although the team had wrangled for months over the proposal, almost no one at the table—including me—expected it to see daylight. I was so skeptical about the politics that I was reluctant to even broach the subject in City Hall. But I felt I had to see the idea fleshed out.

Both Silver and Kansagra were there because Andy Goodman had just reorganized the Division of Health Promotion and Disease Prevention. Silver kept generating creative ideas, but she also continued to upset others in the agency. With my agreement, Goodman created a unit for policy development, with Silver in charge, and another that merged chronic disease prevention with tobacco control, with Kansagra in charge. I hoped the reorganization would play to Silver's strengths, but she was very unhappy with it. Soon after the meeting she left the agency, and we lost one of our best thinkers.

Kansagra and Kennelly, who had become the department's junk food expert, spoke for the group. They stressed that for years health leaders, from the U.S. surgeon general to Michelle Obama, had asked restaurants to voluntarily rein in their monstrous portion sizes—and failed. If restaurants wouldn't restore human-size portions of this dangerous product on their own, they argued, we were obligated to set a reasonable limit. Despite what critics would say, appropriate cup sizes would not affect personal choice; nothing in the rule would prevent people from buying and drinking as much as they want.

The concept was simple, but as always, the details became very messy. The idea would have to run the gauntlet of City Hall, the Board of Health, the press, the soda companies, the restaurants, and the courts, so at every turn there were practical, political, and legal risks. The second-guessers would scrutinize, debate, and attack even the smallest decision. We needed strong reasons to defend each choice.

The rule would apply to drinks with added caloric sweetener that delivered more than 25 calories in 8 ounces. That would allow unlimited portions of pure fruit juices (which had nutritional value and were rarely sold in huge portions) and some new teas that had just a hint of sweetener.

Kennelly proposed to limit the sizes of bottles and cans to 12 ounces, which matched our standards for government vending machines. Even though that feels like a small portion of soda to many Americans these days, 12 ounces was plenty. It delivers more than 8 teaspoons of sugar, which according to the American Heart Association is at the upper limit of what men should consume and more than what women should consume in an entire day. But what about cups filled at soda fountains? As much as a third of the volume of a cup could be ice—something I later verified at a local McDonald's. Kennelly proposed raising the limit for cups to 16 ounces.

I stopped her there. Ice was variable; when you filled your 16-ounce cup at a fountain, you didn't need to add any ice at all. The soda companies, reporters, and lawyers would attack the rule as ridiculous if we had different limits for different containers. Make it 16 ounces for any container, I said. I also hoped that the bigger size might take some of the edge off the attacks.

Drinks containing alcohol would sink us into an entirely different regulatory morass. If a sugary drink was defined as having "added sweetener," 32-ounce steins of beer would be allowed, but mega-size daiquiris wouldn't. That sounded inconsistent. People knocking back daiquiris a quart at a time were risking more than diabetes, but that wasn't the point of the rule. Ultimately, the lawyers ended that conversation. The state alcohol law preempted local governments from doing nearly anything on alcohol. If we included any alcoholic drinks, we'd lose in court. Our rule would have to allow mega-margaritas.

Only later did my chief of staff Kelly Christ pose a tougher question. What about drinks made of milk? McDonald's had milk shakes, and Starbucks had Frappuccinos that walloped consumers with calories. But our health department encouraged people to drink *more* milk for the calcium and vitamin D. Milk-based drinks made up less than 3 percent of the drinks that people ordered at chain restaurants—too small a fraction to be very important. Drawing lines when writing a policy in a complex world always forces choices that appear irrational. We should draw it where the studies on obesity were pointing to, I said. Those studies focused on soda and fruit-flavored drinks—essentially sugar water—not on milk-based drinks. That meant we would allow big milk shakes.

We spent very little time debating what later became our biggest public relations problem: where the rule would apply. The 16-ounce cap would apply in all "food service establishments" that had permits from the health department: the city's 24,000 restaurants, cafeterias, and snack counters (including those at baseball stadiums and movie theaters), as well as outdoor food carts and food trucks. Those were the businesses that we regulated, that our sanitarians inspected, and that were covered by the city health code. Those were the businesses that followed our trans fat rule. Grocery stores, on the other hand, were regulated by New York State, which preempts the Board of Health. For the most part, that distinction fit well with a portion limit. Restaurants sold soda for one person to drink at one meal. Grocery stores sold soda in 2- and 3-liter bottles, but those bottles were to take home, share, and drink over time. Unfortunately, some stores licensed as groceries—like convenience stores—also sold "grab and go" bottles that people drank immediately. Our rule would not stop them from selling bottles larger than 16 ounces, and when a convenience store was next door to a restaurant, that looked inconsistent.

Although the rule applied to every restaurant, from the neighborhood pizza joint to the Four Seasons, the impact was almost entirely on chains like McDonald's and Subway, where most drinks sold were bigger than 16 ounces. A small fraction of the independent restaurants sold drinks larger than that, and those were mostly delis that sold 20-ounce bottles but also carried 12-ounce cans. The "small business" independents would barely notice the rule.

Tom Merrill was firm that the Board of Health had the authority to write the rule. The health code micromanaged nearly everything that happened in restaurants, such as how long food could be kept at room temperature and what kind of materials cutting boards could be made of. As long as we had a strong health justification for every provision of the rule, it should stand up in court. "To me," Merrill said later, "it was always about 'Hey look, you're a restaurant. This is how you're going to serve this product.'"

Kansagra and Kennelly estimated that the portion cap could save 2,400 calories per person a year in New York City. That may seem small—a little over half a pound per person per year—but it was nearly one-third of the 1 to 2 pounds per year that New Yorkers on average were gaining. More important, those extra pounds didn't fall fairly across New York City. Blacks, Latinos, the poor, and genetically predisposed people were gaining much more weight than others. Saving an average of 2,400 calories per New Yorker every year would be big—not as big as the impact of a penny-per-ounce soda tax but bigger than our estimated impact of the SNAP rule change.

Political debates can turn on metaphors. Susan Kansagra's staff looked for other examples of government regulating portion sizes, and found them. Twenty-six regulated the sizes of containers of beer. Most states' laws were meant to permit fair competition in the beer market, not to reduce beer drinking. But two states actually set upper limits for containers of beer: Florida set a cap at 32 ounces and Alabama at 16 ounces.

As Kansagra and Kennelly wrapped up, I saw a ray of hope. Simple policy concepts often crash on the rocks of practicality. It had taken them months, but my team had made the portion cap practical.

• • •

Deputy Mayor Linda Gibbs had become keenly interested in obesity. In early 2012 she convened a multiagency task force to plan how to respond but was a little disappointed that their first ideas felt small. That gave me an opening on the portion cap if I wanted it.

I spent a weekend debating with myself. If the rule were to survive the political and legal obstacle course, it would shine a light on the soda companies' dangerous portion sizes, slow the epidemic, and possibly establish a whole new approach to obesity. Mayor Bloomberg had hired me to generate big ideas for big health problems, and this was one. On the minus side, the soda companies would attack us ferociously, and the press would stoke the controversy. If we lost, and maybe even if we won, our wounds might be large.

I didn't for a moment view the portion cap as interfering with personal choice, because people could order and drink as much as they want, but I was hung up on whether it was an unfair burden to businesses. Then it hit me: not only could customers *buy* two cups at a time, businesses could *sell* two cups at a time. Restaurants could bundle, listing as a single menu item a 32-ounce "large" soda, as long as they delivered it in two 16-ounce cups. That would be a trivial workaround for businesses in return for slowing a killer epidemic. And the beauty was that the portion studies suggested that rule would work anyway, because the psychological default setting would still be one cup of 16 ounces. On this one, I thought, it was better to go down swinging then get caught looking.

"We heard you wanted bigger ideas," I said to Linda Gibbs, sitting at one of the tables overlooking Bloomberg's Bull Pen. "Well, here's a big idea."

"Uh-oh," she said.

· · ·

Not long afterward, sitting in a conference room in City Hall, I made the case to Mayor Bloomberg. Under the watchful eyes of the 1800s-era New York State governors whose portraits hung on the walls, I went through the research on portion sizes and the refilling-soup-bowl study. I also showed him a 1950s-era ad that shows a woman pouring Coke from a tall bottle at a table with three place settings. "Serves 3 over ice—nice!," the caption read. "Big 16 oz size." A short time ago, I argued, Coke advertised a 16-ounce bottle as big enough for a family of three, so how could it be wrong to limit *single* portions to that size?

Bloomberg immediately thought about it from the restaurants' point of view. They should just shrink their drinks to 16 ounces and charge the same amount, he said. Could restaurants offer a buy-one-get-one-free in

16-ounce cups? They could, I said, and the rule would still work. Why don't we regulate grocery stores just as we regulate restaurants? he asked. Preemption, I said.

I could see that he was seriously considering the idea. Like Frieden with the Smoke-Free Air Act a decade earlier, I thought I owed him a little warning. "This will be controversial," I offered. He laughed. "Oh, you figured that out?"

And then he asked for time to think about it.

· · ·

On May 22, 2012, we sent the draft portion rule to the city's Law Department for vetting, and the next day I opened an e-mail that made my heart sink. A reporter from the *Post* had called our press office to say had heard from an inside-government source that we planned to regulate portion sizes for sugary drinks. Reporters often said they had information that they really didn't as a way of prying out more, so I wasn't sure what this reporter knew, but he had hit the topic dead center. We couldn't deny that we were considering a portion cap to him and then announce the rule to the city soon afterward. We had to either kill the idea or announce it.

The scramble to respond brought in the City Hall press office, which was united in hating the idea. To those whose job it was to get flattering stories about the administration, the basic concept looked awful—heavy-handed, nanny-state stuff—and the details even worse. They were upset that someone would be able to buy a 20-ounce bottle of soda from a bodega but not from the deli next door. Or worse, someone could get a giant "Big Gulp" at a 7-Eleven store, which was licensed as a grocery. There were only a few dozen 7-Elevens in New York City, compared to 24,000 licensed food service establishments, so the health impact was negligible, but the symbolism mattered. The press office begged Howard Wolfson to kill the idea, but it was too late. Wolfson also strongly opposed the idea and had argued forcefully against it, but by now the mayor was firm.

Early the next week we met with Wolfson to strategize on the press and the politics. He was boiling over. "How many industries do you guys want to take on?" he yelled. "The restaurants, the soda industry, the movie theaters, the stadiums? . . . Do you know how much money they can throw at this?" He looked around the conference table. "How many people are there in this room?" He counted and then stopped, having made his point. All those industries versus seven of us.

The next day Bloomberg did exclusive interviews with reporters from the *Post*, which the press office had promised in return for their holding the story for a few days, and the *Times*. "Obesity is a nationwide problem," the mayor told the *Times* reporter, "and all over the United States, public health officials are wringing their hands saying 'Oh, this is terrible.' New York City is not about wringing your hands; it's about doing something." For the interviews, Kelly Christ had arranged on the conference table soda cups in sizes ranging from 7 to 64 ounces, then stacked in front of each cup pyramids of sugar cubes showing how much sugar each one held. Even the stack of nine sugar cubes in front of the 7-ounce cup was impressive. The pyramid in front of the 64-ounce cup from KFC was a stunning 12 rows high and contained 87 sugar cubes. In pictures that flew around the globe, Bloomberg is standing behind the stacks, looking feisty.

The *Times* headline was "NEW YORK PLANS TO BAN SALE OF BIG SIZES OF SUGARY DRINKS." The *Post* called the rule a "limit," and the *Journal* a "restriction," but after the *Times* used the word *ban*, the terrible label stuck.

When those stories hit, the media exploded. News outlets acted as if we literally planned to ban soda. The next day so many reporters wanted interviews that Howard Wolfson, Linda Gibbs, and I had to lead an impromptu press conference in the Blue Room to respond to all of them at once. At the last minute we decided to re-create the sugar-cube display, so while a posse of reporters pressed against the door, Kelly Christ (now eight months pregnant) patiently restacked the pyramids.

Once we opened the door, the press packed the room. Photographers sprawled on the floor to get pictures of the sugar cubes. Reporters jumped out of their chairs and shouted questions, the topics of which ranged from bike helmets to National Doughnut Day. When we finished, reporters rushed the front of the room for more. One reporter from a Spanish-language television station breathlessly asked me who would be allowed to order two portions. "It would have to be two persons, right?" No, I assured her. Under the rule, one person could order two—or even more—drinks.

Mayor Bloomberg went on the national media outlets. "Obesity is the only public health issue in this country that's getting worse," he said on NBC. On ABC, he pointed to a "medium"-size cup and told Diane Sawyer, "That was the size of the popcorn I used to get, not the drink." In turn, she asked him about the nicknames "Nanny Mike" and "Soda Scrooge." I took the local television interviews. As I was waiting to go on one morning show, I overheard two employees talking about the rule. One liked the "soda ban" because "people are idiots." Her co-worker apparently disagreed; she followed by asking, without a trace of embarrassment, "How do you get through a whole movie?"

The aftershocks rumbled for days. The papers did man-on-the-street stories. Editorial boards and columnists weighed in: the *Times* editors hated it ("a ban too far" and "too much nannying") and foodie columnist Mark Bittman loved it (sodas are "not food"). On the popular daytime talk show *The View,* Barbara Walters weighed in for it and Whoopi Goldberg against. The late-night comics reveled in it. Stephen Colbert carried out an *Of Mice and Men*–like mercy killing of a five-foot-tall "Drinkee." Jon Stewart hammered on the subject for days, yelling that the rule "combines the draconian government overreach that people love with the lack of results that they expect!" The stories bounced around the globe. A friend of mine, traveling in a small city in Indonesia, was told, "I hear that your mayor wants to ban soda!"

The mayoral candidates were forced to take sides. Christine Quinn came out against the rule, as did rivals Bill Thompson and John Liu. Manhattan borough president Scott Stringer declared in favor. Bill de Blasio, then the public advocate, called me with a few staff on the line and, after probing with a few careful questions, announced for the rule.

Pollsters took the city's pulse. One found that, instead of showing the

60 percent support we had gotten for "limiting the size of sugar-sweet-ened drinks" on an earlier survey, New Yorkers opposed the "soda ban" by 51 to 46 percent.

Howard Wolfson led the charge to get our side of the story in the press. Staff from City Hall and the health department drummed up dozens of approving statements—from people as wide-ranging as Alec Baldwin, Bill Clinton, and Judy Collins—and e-mailed them to reporters daily. The press team organized media events, each with its own message. In one, Mayor Bloomberg was flanked by a pack of white-coated doctors to ring alarms about the crisis of obesity and diabetes in the Bronx. In another, the mayor brandished an endorsement by Weight Watchers to show that the rule would help the millions of New Yorkers struggling to lose weight.

Too often, though, we played defense. Weren't we interfering with personal freedoms? The truth, which rarely came through, was that customers *already* had no choice in soda sizes. No one could buy an 8-ounce cup of soda at McDonald's. At some movie theaters in New York, the smallest size drink for sale was a quart. Someone other than the customer was deciding what size cups to stock, and that someone worked for a corporation that only wanted to sell more soda.

In the tobacco policy battles, Tom Frieden had gone on offense, attacking the tobacco companies as greedy murderers. But Wolfson—reflecting Bloomberg's sentiments—held firm that we would not attack the soda companies. We had no beef with Coke or Pepsi. We were doing this only because portion sizes had gotten out of hand and we had an obligation to answer a health crisis.

We had caught the soda companies by surprise, but after a pause they hit back hard. Their PR firm created a new front group called New Yorkers for Beverage Choices, which put billboards on the backs of soda delivery trucks, with an athletic figure in silhouette defiantly raising a large cup, next to the words "DON'T LET BUREAUCRATS TELL YOU WHAT SIZE BEVERAGE TO BUY." They ran radio spots with "Noo Yawk"–accented actors saying "This is about protecting our freedom of choice," and video ads asking "Are we gonna let the mayor tell us what size beverage to buy? If we let 'em get away with this, where will it end?" They flew banners attacking the rule from airplanes over Coney Island.

They mailed letters to hundreds of thousands of New Yorkers, asking them to sign and return enclosed cards opposing our rule. They organized a "Million Big Gulp March" on City Hall steps, attended by some fifty people, many wearing matching T-shirts saying "I PICKED OUT MY BEVERAGE ALL BY MYSELF." There, under a banner showing a Statue of Liberty–like figure, City Council members and a Teamsters leader rallied the group with words like *tyranny* and *freedom*. For all that, Howard Wolfson thought it could have been worse. "Look, they didn't run TV ads," he said later. "These are companies that are worth many, many billions of dollars."

Five days after the story broke, I testified to City Council at what was supposed to be a routine budget hearing and was pummeled by council members. One complained about the portion rule's "arbitrariness" because we hadn't regulated the sizes of candy bars or beer. Another council member called the "piecemeal" policy "insulting to our intelligence" because it didn't address French fries and hamburgers. A third member, sitting behind a large soda cup, called the rule unfair because "90 percent" of the parents who go to movie theaters buy one large sugary drink and share it to "feed their families" while saving costs. After the hearing, as the council members filed out, they were warmly greeted by the lobbyist for Coca-Cola.

When we tried to rally supporters, we saw how deeply embedded the soda companies are in our society. One obesity researcher whose support we solicited turned us down because she believed her endorsement might jeopardize her ability to get grants. The head of a health insurance company, which would benefit financially if people stayed healthy, told me that he couldn't support the portion rule because he would "catch hell" from his clients, the bottling companies.

Inside the health department, my team was actually heartened by the soda companies' nuclear response. Susan Kansagra said later, "We knew they were out there, they were probably spending a lot of money, and we felt that was good because that meant they were really scared about the impact of this proposal." Maybe their overreaction really did mean that we had hit on a great idea. But with all their firepower, it also meant that they might win.

．　．　．

The Board of Health meeting on Tuesday, June 12, was scheduled to start at ten a.m., but the media trucks began arriving in front of the health department's new building in Queens at five. The meeting room was sterile, long and narrow, and had a glass wall on the long side, so onlookers in the hallway could watch the board members as if they were in a large fishtank. That day the members sat behind folding tables arranged in an L shape, some alongside and some facing a space set aside for the cameras. The photographers spilled beyond the space, though, with some lying on the floor and others peeking their lenses over the shoulders of competitors. The rest of the room was filled with rows of chairs packed with print reporters, people in dark suits who looked like lawyers or lobbyists, and health department staff.

The soda companies and the press assumed that the board was a rubber stamp for the mayor, but the members were in fact independent health experts. They were appointed by the mayor but confirmed by the City Council; they served fixed six-year terms and could be removed only based on proof of misconduct or inability to function. Of the eleven board members, seven were doctors, three were health care managers, and one was a professor of public health. None knew Bloomberg personally, were part of any political organization, or had any political ambitions. The board rarely rejected a proposed rule from the health department, but after seeing how affected people or businesses reacted to a rule during the required public comment period, they or the health department often altered the rule.

A law prevented board members from conversing about proposed rules outside open meetings, and Tom Merrill always insisted that we scrupulously obey. A week before the meeting, we had sent the members the portion rule and a memo explaining the reasoning behind it. Other than that, until the meeting, the board members knew only what they had seen in the press. I had no idea how they would react.

Susan Kansagra sat facing them at the witness table, with Maura Kennelly at her side, looking small and a little nervous. After she summarized the rule and its rationale, showing slides on the video screens wrapping around the long room, board members took turns asking polite questions. They wanted to understand the 16-ounce cutoff, how the rule would handle ice in a cup, and diet drinks. Bruce Vladeck, a gruff health care systems consultant who once ran the federal Health Care Financing Administration, asked about capping portion sizes for popcorn at movie theaters. Deepu Gowda, an earnest young internist from Columbia University, asked about taxing soda instead. Mike Phillips, a public health physician from New York University, sounded skeptical. He asked what was unique about sugary drinks. What about hamburgers and French fries—hadn't their portion sizes grown too? And why didn't the rule apply to convenience stores? When Kansagra explained why, he asked politely, "Is that fair?"

Only one board member, Brooklyn primary care doctor Sixto Caro, seemed clearly against the rule. He worried out loud that it would somehow increase taxes for small businesses. "When a consumer buys 16 ounces, they pay 8.25 percent. If they buy a second one, they pay more taxes. And the small business has to pay those taxes. . . . Why are we targeting the low-income small businesses instead of the big companies?" But at the end of the questioning, the board voted unanimously to publish the rule for public comment.

• • •

The day before the board meeting, Coca-Cola CEO Muhtar Kent had asked Bloomberg to meet. Three days later he flew to New York City with Steven Cahillane, the CEO of Coca-Cola Refreshments, its North American bottling company, and two others. Howard Wolfson, Linda Gibbs, and I joined the mayor to meet them at the dining room table at Gracie Mansion, over a linen tablecloth and cans of Coke Zero.

Kent, the son of a Turkish consul-general who was born in New York

City, has a broad chest, impeccable grooming, an accent that reflects his British education, and a big winning smile. After chatting for ten minutes with Bloomberg about the depression and the teetering financial system in Europe, he made his case. "We are a marketing company and a hydration company," he said. "We are not perfect," but his company was trying to do its part to solve the obesity problem. It was "not an accident" that sales of diet beverages had risen to 30 percent of the market. Now, though, our rule was killing them. He had just come from Europe, where everyone was saying, "'I hear Mayor Bloomberg is banning your product in New York City.' Even though we know that's not exactly what you are proposing, that is the perception." To have this iconic product, the global symbol of America, banned by the city that is the symbol of America was ruining its image. Instead of fighting each other, we should work together, he said. We could accomplish so much more if we did—Coke with its ability to influence the consumer and Mayor Bloomberg with his global reputation in health.

Cahillane, the son of a New York firefighter with roots in Ireland, had a thin face, sandy hair, and an appealing directness about him. He was a manager who had worked his way up through the beer business. Coke had done a pilot project in the Bronx, he said, that had led to a 10 percent increase in the sales of diet beverages and a 2.5 percent decrease in the sales of full-calorie sodas. That showed what they could do.

Kent proposed to take the Bronx pilot project citywide if we agreed to withdraw the rule for a year. It would have a greater impact on calorie consumption in New York City, he said, than our rule would. Dr. Farley could model the impact to verify that that was true, he said, opening his arms to show that he had nothing to hide. And he was sure that if we agreed, he could bring Pepsi along with the plan.

It was the only time I ever saw Mike Bloomberg look uncomfortable. He was a businessman before he was mayor, and he didn't like opposing another businessman. He was concerned about obesity, he said. But two people on the Coke board had already spoken to him about this. He wanted to work with Coke. And then he asked Howard Wolfson to follow up on Coke's offer.

That set off some frantic negotiations. Cahillane came back to New York a few days later with a concrete proposal. Coke would ramp up its promotion of diet products in grocery and convenience stores, introduce smaller bottles and cans in groceries (without eliminating the larger sizes), introduce 12-ounce cup sizes in restaurants that didn't already offer them, and replace some of the full-calorie options on restaurant soda fountains with diet sodas. Over the next three years, he claimed, that would lead to a 12 percent reduction in the calories that New Yorkers got from sugary drinks. And he would throw in funding to support a few physical activity programs.

After spending some hours with spreadsheets, I was convinced that Cahillane's proposal actually had the potential to cut sugary drink consumption substantially. It was tempting to consider a big agreement using the power of Coca-Cola to reduce sugary drink consumption. But the Coke people knew so much more about the business than we did. I was worried that we could be hoodwinked.

I wrote my own balance sheet. On the plus side, Coke's offer would affect more distribution channels than our policy, which affected restaurants only. The city might indeed see a health benefit, and the political pressure and the press noise would disappear.

But the minus side was long. Coke would have to get the other soda companies to agree. Coke hadn't shown us any hard data from its Bronx pilot or offered any numbers to measure progress. We would be completely dependent on the corporation's actions, with no way to verify what it was doing. In another eighteen months, we would be out of power; if Coke's plan was going off track, even if we knew it, we'd be helpless. Most of the changes the company proposed were ones that it was already making in response to public pressure on obesity—or should have been making. And dropping our rule would eliminate, probably forever, the policy tool of limiting portion sizes as a way of fighting obesity.

I went through my thinking with Howard Wolfson and Linda Gibbs. Then we got back together with Cahillane and tried to discuss other portion-reducing possibilities, but the conversation quickly went downhill. Cahillane complained that soda was only a tiny part of the diet, and that we were only going after Coke because it was such a high-profile target. I disagreed; we were attacking soda (not just Coke) because of studies linking it to the massive obesity epidemic. Without getting rid of large portion sizes, I said, there was no guarantee that we would ever see a fall in consumption. Coke couldn't possibly take away any portion sizes, Cahillane said, because that implied "Coke is bad." If we didn't accept this offer, he would take it to another city, which would reap the benefits that New York City had turned down, and Coke would fight the portion rule tooth and nail.

17

"The NSRI's success is far from guaranteed."

On February 11, 2013, I stood in City Hall's ornate Outer Ceremonial Room with representatives of seven food companies, waiting for Mayor Bloomberg. It was the same room in which we had gathered three years earlier to unveil the companies' promises to cut salt in their food. Now we would cheer what they had achieved.

But I wasn't sure whether we could call the entire project a success. After the launch in early 2010, we had hoped a swell of other companies would join the parade, but only a few had done so. It wasn't clear if enough companies had enlisted to make a meaningful difference. In 2012 the Center for Science in the Public Interest checked the nutrition labels of 480 packaged and restaurant foods, comparing the sodium content in 2011 to that of 2005. Sodium levels had fallen in 43 percent of food items and risen in 33 percent. On average, they fell by 3.5 percent in packaged foods but rose by 2.6 percent in restaurant foods.

It was still early, but that hardly felt like a victory. By the fall of 2012, most of the food industry seemed to have realized it could safely ignore us. Sonia Angell and I wrote a paper in the *American Journal of Public Health* trying to warn the companies that by doing nothing they risked a heavier government hand. "The NSRI's success is far from guaranteed," we wrote. "It is unlikely that the current number of company commitments will substantially alter the sodium composition of our nation's food supply. . . . If this process does not lead to meaningful industry-wide reductions, it justifies the call for regulation recommended by the IOM committee."

Just as this article appeared, though, Christine Curtis was reviewing the first reports from the companies that had signed on. After she verified the data, "we were really excited." Twenty-one of the twenty-four companies that had publicly promised to lower sodium by 2012 had met their targets. They had done what many other food companies had said was impossible, and they had done it quickly.

Curtis noticed something else exciting. She and her staff labored for many long hours updating their food databases with nutrition data. As they typed numbers into their computers, they noted that some companies that had spurned the NSRI were nonetheless reporting lower sodium levels. Apparently, while they had been afraid of making a public commitment, they had quietly made changes anyway.

The companies that had made public promises still deserved a public thanks. So I stood with representatives of Kraft, Mondelēz (a global company that had split from Kraft), Mars, Goya, Subway, Fresh Direct (an online grocer), and LiDestri (a regional maker of pasta sauces). As we waited, we talked about salt. Because other food companies had complained so bitterly, I was curious about how the winners had pulled it off. The vice president for R&D at Kraft, talked excitedly about substituting potassium chloride for sodium chloride in a food laboratory, sometimes adding other ingredients to mask the potassium's bitterness, and testing the changes to meet a taste profile. But a manager from Goya, a much smaller company that marketed products mainly to Hispanics, shrugged. Goya had just put less salt in the beans.

Then Bloomberg arrived. He thanked them all and led us to the Blue Room to face the cameras. "Today I'm pleased to announce that twenty-one major food companies have reached [our] 2012 sodium reduction goals," he said. "This group is no small potatoes: it includes some of the biggest packaged food companies, restaurants, and food retailers in the country, if not the world. . . . The products they're making healthier are some of America's most beloved and iconic foods."

The changes would touch the lives of millions. Kraft had cut sodium in sliced American cheese by 18 percent. Mondelēz had taken out 33 percent of the sodium in Teddy Grahams. Subway reduced the sodium in Bloomberg's favorite Italian BMT sandwich by 27 percent. Mars had taken 15 percent of the sodium out of its Uncle Ben's flavored rice mixes. And Heinz had met its promise to cut sodium in ketchup by 15 percent. Only three of twenty-four companies that made commitments for 2012 failed to meet them: Hostess, which had gone bankrupt, and Boar's Head and Bertucci's, which were still trying.

We got the press attention that we wanted, as upbeat stories ran in news outlets across the country. But even the companies that wanted the public recognition were edgy about what Mayor Bloomberg would say. They didn't want to broadcast that they were putting less salt in their foods, because they were afraid that it would hurt sales. Susan Kansagra had stopped off at a grocery store that morning to buy Teddy Grahams, Heinz ketchup, and Kraft American cheese in case the reporters wanted to take shots of those foods, but the companies vetoed photos. They didn't want pictures circulating on the web attracting comments that their name-brand products would now taste bad.

. . .

The more progress we made, the louder the noises from the scientific doubters. And unfortunately, the news media helped them sow confusion.

In 2011 the *Journal of the American Medical Association* published two papers that seemed to show higher death rates in people taking in low amounts of sodium. Both used data from other studies that were designed to answer different research questions; the authors were engaging in after-the-fact "data dredging." Both were quickly and roundly criticized as flawed. In particular, the way the authors had measured sodium intake was unreliable. More important, their findings looked like "reverse causation"—that is, people in the study may have been on low-sodium diets because they were already sick with heart or kidney disease. It wouldn't be surprising, then, if the people taking in less salt were more likely to die within the next few years. But the two studies muddied the issue outside the medical world. Articles appeared like the one in the *Times,* which ran the headline "LOW-SALT DIET INEFFECTIVE, STUDY FINDS. DISAGREEMENT ABOUNDS."

At about the same time, a different research group published a prominent "meta-analysis" of trials of low-sodium diets. A meta-analysis combines data from many other studies; this one merged data from seven. The authors claimed to see "no strong evidence that salt reduction reduced all-cause mortality" in people who didn't already have congestive heart failure. And they saw an increased death rate in people on low-salt diets who already had congestive heart failure—a finding that came from just one of the seven studies they had combined. The authors admitted that even with the combined data, their study did not contain nearly enough people to draw any conclusions about low-salt diets in typical people. And they wrote that "our findings are consistent with the belief that salt reduction is beneficial" in people who didn't already have advanced heart disease. Nonetheless Michael Alderman (the doctor who had warned against low-salt diets in 2010) trumpeted the meta-analysis, writing that "this scholarly review . . . challenges the assumptions of a relation between sodium intake and CVD [cardiovascular disease] and its policy implications."

From there, the story gathered momentum. *Scientific American* ran an article titled "It's Time to End the War on Salt" and subtitled, "The zealous drive by politicians to limit our salt intake has little basis in science." That triggered a story in the *Wall Street Journal* attacking us directly. "Mayor Michael Bloomberg's war against salt has put him in the cross hairs of medical researchers," the story read. "A new analysis by an internationally respected research body has cast doubt on the city's claims about the perils of a salty diet." Other newspapers went all the way. The U.K.'s *Daily Express* headline read "NOW SALT IS SAFE TO EAT."

That was quite a transformation. The story went from the meta-analysis's authors writing that salt reduction for most people was probably beneficial, to reporters writing exactly the opposite. The pivot seemed to have been Alderman's editorial. Alderman, the former adviser to the industry's Salt Institute, wrote frequently that reducing salt intake might be dangerous, which he could do whenever he wanted to because he edited his own journal.

Two years later the story got even fishier when the authors of the meta-analysis retracted their paper. They had learned a disturbing story about the researchers behind the only one of their seven studies show-ing an increase in mortality from a low-salt diet. The lead author of the suspicious paper was listed as working for Wegmans pharmacy in Ithaca, New York. He and his coauthors were suspected of using data from the same patients in two different studies, then combining them in their own meta-analysis. Either of those would be considered scientific malprac-tice. When a journal committee investigating asked to see their raw data, the researchers claimed the data no longer existed because of a computer crash. That was enough for the investigating committee. After their suspi-cious trial was removed from the larger meta-analysis, the results changed sharply, with lower sodium diets now leading to fewer heart attacks and strokes. In the wake of the retraction, Alderman did not retract his edito-rial, and neither *Scientific American* nor the *Journal* corrected its article.

Around the time the meta-analysis was published, the CDC asked the Institute of Medicine to review recent studies and recommend how much Americans should cut their salt intake. The IOM committee recon-firmed that people should take in less sodium, but then got squeamish about exactly how much. The committee was comfortable with the less-than-2,300 mg recommendations in the current guidelines for healthy people. But it wasn't willing to endorse the recommendations that people with certain health risks (people over fifty, blacks, and those with high blood pressure or diabetes) should go further, cutting back to less than 1,500 mg per day. It ducked, claiming "not sufficient evidence" to address that secondary question.

Michael Alderman jumped on the IOM report too, saying it "has changed the paradigm through which the issue of sodium intake can be addressed. The default position is no longer 'lower is always better.'" Reporters also interpreted the review as a radical change in scientific thinking. *The Washington Post*'s headline was "STUDY QUESTIONS EFFORTS TO SLASH INTAKE OF SALT," and *The New York Times* wrote that the IOM review "undercuts years of public health warnings." In their details, the stories didn't misrepresent the IOM findings, but most people reading only the headlines would think that experts were now saying that salt was not bad for you after all.

This may sound like trivial squabbling among scientists, but many lives were at stake. The scientific facts on salt mattered to the two-thirds of Americans over age sixty who, like Sylvia Birnbaum, had high blood pressure, and to the hundreds of thousands who were dying every year from heart attacks and strokes caused by hypertension. People affiliated with the salt manufacturers were claiming—against decades of evidence—that salt is not bad for you, and the press was serving as their megaphone. Unfortunately, the default course in our democracy is inaction. To prevent progress, the critics don't have to prove anything. Like climate change deniers, all they have to do is introduce doubt.

The most important fact, which was lost in the *Post* and *Times* articles, was that 90 percent of Americans took in more sodium—usually much more—than even the higher recommendation of 2,300 mg. It didn't matter whether the healthy target was 1,500 mg or 2,300 mg. Even if New York City's initiative met its ambitious long-term goal of dropping sodium intake by 20 percent, the average American would still be consuming about 2,700 mg. Nearly every expert—other than those affiliated with the Salt Institute—agreed that making that change would save many lives.

· · ·

In late 2011 the FDA showed flickers of life. The agency released a "docket," or an invitation for anyone to comment, on "effective strategies for sustainable and meaningful reduction of sodium in foods." The docket didn't obligate the FDA to do anything specific, but it meant that the agency wanted to do something on salt.

If we had any hope for long-term success on salt, we needed action from the FDA, the only agency in the nation with authority over packaged food. I wanted the FDA to simply add its regulatory clout to the sodium targets that we had already developed. Lynn Silver, as always, had ideas of her own. She wanted the FDA to put warning labels on food packages if sodium was especially high. When the FDA held a hearing on the docket, Christine Curtis traveled to Washington to tell our story. The hearing brought out the other major players on salt, too. Health experts praised the FDA for finally turning its attention to the problem. Food companies said they were trying to lower sodium but were hamstrung by their customers. And operatives from the Salt Institute and their paid experts said that cutting salt might kill people.

Then we waited. Christine Curtis heard a rumor that the FDA wanted to create its own voluntary sodium-reduction targets. Then we heard that the White House had bottled even that up. "It was clear that there was a general regulatory paralysis going on" in Obama's White House, said Lynn Silver. It reminded Susan Kansagra of what happened a year earlier, when federal agencies tried to write guidelines to limit the marketing of junk food to children. Even though the guidelines were weak and voluntary, the food industry's friends in Congress strangled the idea.

In the meantime, other countries' governments were acting. Health officials in Canada developed their own sodium reduction plan, asking for advice as they did from Curtis. The Canadians built databases like hers and used a similar process to set national targets for food companies. Curtis also talked with government health officials from Australia and New Zealand as they shaped their salt strategies. Most frustrating to us, many of the food companies negotiating with these British Commonwealth countries were the same global companies that Lynn Silver, Sonia Angell, and Christine Curtis had been meeting with since 2007. They were working on salt with more than one national government, but not with our own.

. . .

At the time of that celebratory press conference with Kraft and Goya, it had been eight years since Silver had first seen the report *Salt: The Forgotten Killer.* In those years, we had succeeded in making salt a little less forgotten. A question that nagged us, though, was how much of the killer the food companies had really taken out.

Curtis had to work around some missing data, especially sales data from Walmart, but she estimated that between 2009 and 2012, the sodium in the U.S. packaged food supply fell by 5 to 6 percent. Among the most important food categories, those showing the biggest changes were breakfast cereal, barbecue sauce, and bread, each down 8 percent, and—a little victory from the meeting in 2009—crackers, down 12 percent. She didn't see any changes in restaurant food, which was no surprise because the restaurants barely spoke to us.

How important were these changes? Even the people who spent much of their lives thinking about salt disagreed. Kansagra called it only "slight progress." On the other hand, a CDC expert told me that if we had actually cut sodium by 6 percent over just three years, "that would be huge," especially after the utter failure over the previous forty years. Curtis also saw the changes much more brightly. The salt reductions in the crackers and bread categories were big, she thought, more than most people ever expected. Also, there was a lag in getting changes into her database, and based on what she was hearing from companies, she expected the fall to continue.

Tom Frieden always demands a "back-of-the-envelope on lives saved," so here it is: a researcher from the University of California at San Francisco estimated that lowering salt intake by 11 percent would prevent between 17,000 and 28,000 deaths per year nationwide. If Curtis's estimates are right, our National Salt Reduction Initiative would reduce Americans' total sodium intake by about a fourth of that. That is, every year in the United States it might prevent 6,000 deaths from heart attack and stroke. Six thousand is more than twice the number of people who died in the 9/11 attacks. It's only people in public health who consider a number like that to be embarrassingly small.

18

"This is an attack on
small business."

In July 2012, six weeks after the meetings with Coke at Gracie
Mansion, the Board of Health was back in the health department's glass-walled room for a public hearing on the proposed soda portion limit. This time I counted twenty-two video cameras, and our press office counted seventy-five press outlets. At this meeting, any interested citizen had the opportunity to sit at a folding table in front of the board for three minutes—as an LED timer counted down the seconds—and speak his or her mind; the board members were there only to listen.

Coke did not send representatives. Nor did PepsiCo. Nor did McDonald's, Burger King, KFC, or any other chain restaurant that sold the huge sugary drinks. But the soda industry was amply represented. The industry lobbyists took turns denying that obesity was their clients' fault. Joy Dubost of the National Restaurant Association said that the restaurant industry "plays a positive role reversing the trend of obesity, including adding more healthful options to menus and disclosing nutrition information." A representative of the National Association of Theater Owners argued that "in moderation most things are okay. Well, sales of sugary drinks at movie theaters are just that. They are moderation defined. Why? The average moviegoer in New York City only goes to the theater four times a year." Jim McGreevy of the American Beverage Association was forced to address sugary drinks more head-on. "A substantial body of literature confirms that sugar-sweetened beverages are not a unique driver of obesity rates," he said.

They and the other opponents hit repeatedly on common themes: The rule wouldn't work. The exclusions—alcohol, dairy products, convenience stores—were nonsensical. We should instead fight obesity with education and exercise programs. The rule was an interference with personal freedom. The rule was not just a job killer, it was unfair specifically to small businesses, especially minority-owned ones.

Several City Council members joined the soda companies in attacking the proposal. Daniel Halloran, an aggressive Republican with libertarian leanings who later got convicted in a bribery scandal, was the first to speak. "They came for the cigarettes; I didn't say anything. I didn't smoke. When they came for the MSG, I really didn't care because I didn't order it very often. I am not a big salt eater so I didn't mind when you guys regulated salt. What will the government be telling me next: What time to go to bed? How big my steak should be? How many potato chips I could have?" He was followed by Council members Robert Jackson, an African American, and Melissa Mark-Viverito, a Puerto Rican, who denounced the rule's "adverse economic impact on our communities." Then Joseph Vitta, a hulk of a man and the secretary-treasurer of Teamsters Local 812, warned the board that if sales of soda went down, his union workers would lose jobs.

But the health advocates also had their moments. Walter Willett, the chair of the department of nutrition at the Harvard School of Public Health, warned that "large doses of sugar are metabolically toxic" and said those doses were hitting poor minorities especially hard. Michael Jacobson of the Center for Science in the Public Interest attacked the soda industry more directly, saying that "the freedom to sell supersized junk means little compared to the necessity to protect New Yorkers from the obesity epidemic." Kelly Brownell, a professor and anti-obesity advocate from Yale, said, "The industry behavior on this is . . . stunningly similar to what I saw in the tobacco wars."

And David Jones, a prominent African American civil rights advocate, called the soda companies' behavior "a direct attack on New York's black and brown communities." "I should mention, one hundred years ago, we were fighting a somewhat similar effort, where chalk was being used to add to water and sold to poor mothers as a substitute for milk." And now, he said, the soda companies had "the audacity to equate this whole process to what they describe as the Million Big Gulp March, and it is a takeoff obviously on the Million Man March, an effort that was made to protect particularly black young people and black men. . . . To suddenly make a sham of that, to equate civil rights and the struggle that is occurring in poor neighborhoods, particularly for the young, to this right to sell nonnutritional substances to young people is an outrage."

Toward the end of the hearing, Liz Berman, representing the front group New Yorkers for Beverage Choices, theatrically dropped on the witness table a petition with 91,000 signatures and bags of more than 6,000 postcards opposing the proposal. "The citywide outpouring of opposition to this proposal is testament to the fact that New Yorkers feel that this proposal is arbitrary, it is unfair, and it is ineffective."

But she was followed by Daniel Simon, a bearded, soft-spoken young man who introduced himself as just "a citizen." "And in the interest of full disclosure, nobody is paying me to be here. In fact, I spent $2.25 of my own money to get here on the subway." He had been approached by a man on 42nd Street to sign his name to "fight back against the Bloomberg ban." The man approaching him said he was being paid thirty dollars an hour to collect signatures, and "he told me to e-mail his boss if I wanted a job" doing the same. The man had handed Simon an iPad to sign, but "the full screen was just a field to put my name and digital signature. There was no preamble to the petition even."

· · ·

The board members met again in September 2012 to consider the public comments and to vote on the rule. In advance, they had received a DVD with copies of each of the written comments. There were 32,000 in support and 6,000 in opposition. Although many were from ordinary citizens, the stack made it clear that this war was between health organizations and the soda industry. Unlike comments on most proposed Board of Health rules, virtually none of the criticisms suggested alterations to the rule. The soda companies and their allies wanted only to kill it.

Susan Kansagra had also sent the board members a thirteen-page memo grouping the public comments into themes, with the health department's responses, and now she took thirty minutes at the witness table to go through them. She ended with, "If you look at the other public health measures that have been put in place, things like smoke-free restaurants, restrictions on trans fat, removal of lead in paint, these were also met with opposition from industry as well as the public. And if you look at some of the headlines from a few years ago, they could very easily be written today, but those things are now widely accepted." Because the critics had proposed no changes to the rule, neither did she.

Then the board members got their chance to weigh in. Sandro Galea, an epidemiologist from Columbia University with an elegant, intellectual manner, said that after "I spent many lovely hours" reading the thousands of comments, "I thought the evidence was very clear epidemiologically that behavioral choice drifts to what is available to us, to all humans." And "the argument about choice is also a false argument. . . . As consumers, our choice is already ultimately set by the food service establishment, and all this is doing is creating the bounds of those choices, which is exactly the role of the health department." Lynn Richardson, an emergency room physician, said, "I have to admit I was skeptical prior to hearing the initial proposal and presentations. But I found the arguments made by the department and in support of the proposal to be convincing, even compelling, and those of the opponents . . . they were really not persuasive at all." She and other board members said they were moved by seeing in their practice so many people, especially blacks and Latinos from poor neighborhoods, suffering from obesity and diabetes. Joel Forman, a pediatrician who saw many children from East Harlem and the South Bronx, said, "The problems we deal with every day are obesity, obesity, asthma, obesity, asthma." He said, "I can't imagine the board not acting on some other problem that was killing five thousand people a year." Only Sixto Caro differed, again raising the concern about the additional cost of buying two 16-ounce sodas instead of one 32-ounce soda, and criticizing the rule as being "not comprehensive enough."

At the end, all board members except Sixto Caro voted in favor. To give the restaurants and soda companies plenty of time to make changes, the rule would go into effect in six months.

After the vote, Mayor Bloomberg held a triumphant press conference with Bruce Ratner, the developer who was just finishing building the Barclays Center, a sports arena in downtown Brooklyn. Ratner had agreed to voluntarily adopt the 16-ounce limit from the day it would open. When a reporter asked Bloomberg about the soda industry's well-financed opposition, he came back at her. "I've spent $600 million on tobacco control, and I'm looking for another cause. Now how much did you say they were spending again?"

. . .

Coca-Cola made good on both of Steven Cahillane's threats. In October 2012, a month after the Board of Health passed the portion cap, the powerhouse law firm Latham & Watkins, working for the American Beverage Association, sued to block the rule. The ABA was joined in the lawsuit by others that made money from big sodas: the National Restaurant Association (which represents the big chains) and the National Association of Theater Owners of New York State. And they brought along the New York State Coalition of Hispanic Chambers of Commerce, the New York Korean-American Grocers Association, the Soft Drink and Brewery Workers Union, and Local 812 of the Teamsters. The Board of Health did not have the authority to pass the portion rule, their lawyers wrote, and the rule was "arbitrary and capricious in its design and application." The law firm channeled the public relations war into the courtroom, referring to the rule as "The Ban," capitalized, and prominently citing the ninety-thousand-name petition and polls showing that a majority of New Yorkers opposed it.

Coca-Cola brought race into the courtroom too. The corporation's longtime law firm King & Spalding delivered an amicus brief, signed by the NAACP and the Hispanic Federation. These organizations had

"fought long and hard to protect and enliven the voices of their community members in the political system," they wrote. But with the portion
rule, the "Board of Health and unelected appointees, like Commissioner
Farley, circumvented those voices, along with the voice of millions of
New Yorkers, when the board told New Yorkers that it would selectively
and unfairly harm small and minority-owned businesses." The NAACP
had deep ties to Coca-Cola and had recently received tens of thousands of
dollars from Coke for a health education program. The former president
of the Hispanic Federation had just taken a job at Coca-Cola.

Then in November, Cahillane stood with Chicago mayor Rahm
Emanuel and officials from PepsiCo and Dr Pepper Snapple Group to
announce that the soda companies were giving that city $5 million. The
money would go for a wellness competition between city employees in
Chicago and San Antonio. In return, Emanuel promised to kill a proposed sugary drink tax and not pursue a New York City–style portion
cap. Emanuel seemed to blame overweight people for their problems. "If
you basically put aside personal responsibility," the mayor said, "you're
missing the core ingredient for improving health care outcomes." It was
the first of three payoffs that Coke would make to Chicago over the next
nine months. In the second, it gave the city $3 million for nutrition and
exercise classes. In the third, Emanuel put images of Coke products on
50,000 blue household recycling carts bought with $2.6 million from the
Coca-Cola Foundation.

Tom Merrill was, in a way, relieved when he read the legal papers. The
soda companies' line of attack was what he had predicted. It was based on
the 1987 case *Boreali v. Axelrod*, in which the state's Public Health Council, a group of experts answering to the state health commissioner, had
tried to ban smoking in restaurants with more than fifty seats. The state
court of appeals struck down the rule, saying it amounted to legislation,
which only the state legislature could enact. In its opinion, the court laid
down criteria for how future judges could distinguish legislation from
regulations.

Merrill and the rest of the city's lawyers were convinced that the

Boreali decision didn't apply to the New York City Board of Health. Ever since the 1800s, the state legislature had given the board unique authority—often called by the courts "legislative"—to pass rules on health that had the force of law; the Public Health Council didn't have that authority. The board used its authority to manage various crises, like cholera and yellow fever, that the legislature was hopeless at handling. The state's highest court had affirmed this authority in 1868 when the board regulated the slaughtering of cattle, in 1965 when it fluoridated the city's drinking water, and in 1976 when it required landlords to install window guards to protect toddlers from falls. But just in case, Merrill had made sure to draft the portion cap rule to meet the *Boreali* criteria.

The case landed on the desk of Judge Milton Tingling, a fifty-nine-year-old African American from the Washington Heights neighborhood. Judge Tingling was known for his sympathy and patience, but his rulings signaled that he was deeply skeptical of government power. Delayed by mix-ups in the court and by Hurricane Sandy, the case didn't come to him until early 2013. By that time, both legal teams were in a rush to get a decision before the rule went into effect that March.

At the oral argument, Susan Kansagra, watching from the gallery, saw "our folks against this wall of corporate-looking lawyers." Merrill presented the city's argument that the portion rule was rational and within the board's traditional authority. When the other side's lawyers spoke, they got a little overheated. As recounted by the *New York Times*:

> *Mr. Brandt, the industry lawyer, at one point suggested the soda rules would lead to a slippery slope of Orwellian government micromanagement.*
>
> *"What comes next?" Mr. Brandt asked. "Red meat twice a week, but no more? You can buy your bacon and cheese in the morning, but no eggs on it? No jaywalking, because you might get hurt, if you jaywalk?"*
>
> *At this, Justice Tingling, who rarely spoke during the proceedings and betrayed few signs of his thinking on the case, chose to weigh in.*
>
> *"For the record, counsel, jaywalking is illegal," the judge said, smiling. "But I got you."*

. . .

On March 11, 2013, the day before the portion rule was to go into effect, Judge Tingling slapped the Board of Health down hard. The *Boreali* criteria applied to the Board of Health, he ruled, and on those criteria the portion rule failed. But he went far beyond that. The rule was "arbitrary and capricious," he wrote, riddled with "loopholes" like free refills. And even more breathtaking: the Board of Health had the authority to prevent only "communicable, infectious, and pestilent diseases." "To accept the respondents' interpretation of its authority granted to the Board by the New York City Charter would leave its authority to define, create, mandate, and enforce limited only by its own imagination," Tingling concluded. "The Rule would not only violate the separation of powers doctrine, it would eviscerate it. Such an evisceration has the potential to be more troubling than sugar sweetened beverages."

At City Hall, Bloomberg was furious. At the health department, we were horrified. Tingling had done far more damage than just stop the portion rule. His opinion that the board's authority was limited to infectious diseases, if it stood, would destroy its authority to protect New Yorkers from the most important health problems of our time. It meant the board could not have banned trans fat, required calorie labeling, or banned lead in paint. According to Tom Merrill, the ruling "would pretty much have invalidated most of the Department." I could blame the soda companies, the judge—or myself—for that, but regardless, the future of public health in New York City was now in deep trouble.

The city lawyers were just as upset but not despairing. We had a 90 percent chance of winning on appeal, they said—the law was clearly on our side.

I was beginning to take a different lesson. At about the same time, we had a resounding win in an unrelated legal case that the city lawyers thought we were likely to lose. Court decisions appeared to depend entirely on the whims of whatever judge drew the short straw. The *Boreali* criteria were vague enough that a judge could read them whatever way he wanted. This case felt like a crapshoot.

The flood of news stories about the ruling took a different angle, one that was nearly as bad. Tingling's verdict was strictly about which body of government, the Board of Health or the City Council, had the authority to pass a portion limit, but his words were so harsh that they implied that a soda portion limit was morally wrong. That was the tone of the soda companies' PR blitz, and that was the tone that the press now broadcast around the world. The *Times* captured it: "It would have amounted to a tax on the poor, said some. It would have had little effect anyway, noted others, because people would still have been allowed free refills. It was un-American, said others still, for was this not the country of freedom, more or less, of choice?" The polls showed New Yorkers' opinions followed, with support for the "ban" dropping from 46 percent two weeks before the ruling to 39 percent a month after. All told, the judge's decision couldn't have been worse.

Mayor Bloomberg came out defiant. Obesity was "a health crisis," he said to reporters. "People are dying every day. . . . This is about real lives." He fired at Tingling. "The judge is totally in error in the way that he interpreted the law," he said. The city would win on appeal. "Being the first to do something is never easy."

And to show how reasonable the rule was, the City Hall press office organized a press conference next day at Lucky's Café, a closet of a deli in midtown Manhattan. The owner, Greg Anagnostopoulos, had agreed to limit his soda cups to 16 ounces voluntarily. Bloomberg stood amid a pack of supporters, including a doctor, a pastor, Harlem children's advocate Geoffrey Canada, and mayoral candidate Bill de Blasio, and charged forward. "Despite yesterday's temporary setback, I don't think that there is any doubt that the momentum is moving in our direction. . . . While the legal case plays out, the conversation that has started about the dangers of large sugary drinks has prompted many people like Greg to take action." When a reporter asked if he would continue his "anti-obesity crusade" after his term was over, Bloomberg snapped back, "You can take that to the bank."

. . .

The city's appeal in the sugary drink portion cap case took place in June 2013, in the ornate Beaux Arts courtroom of the appellate division on the corner of Madison Avenue and 25th Street. This time the case was heard by a panel of five judges.

It was ugly. The soda companies' lawyer was as smooth as silk. The judges, for the most part, quietly heard him out as he characterized the rule as a loophole-filled, irrational power grab by the Board of Health. The city's lawyer, Fay Ng, was steeped in the law but, unlike Tom Mer- rill, didn't work in the health department and hadn't spent months study- ing the health details. She had barely opened her mouth before the judges pounced. How did the Board of Health decide on 16 ounces? Wasn't that arbitrary? What was the justification for including sweetened teas but not milk shakes? What nutritional value did milk shakes have? "They didn't even wait for her response," said Susan Kansagra, who sat cringing in the gallery. "They were just *boom boom boom* asking questions." The hearing "was less about the legal case than it was about the policy and what was in the press," said Maura Kennelly.

The courtroom had become a mirror for the public debate, and the public debate—shaped by the PR barrage of the soda companies—was leaning hard against us. "We definitely lost the messaging," said Tom Merrill. "It became this liberty interest."

"And if you can't get past that as a judge or as a panel of judges," said Kennelly, "then that lens is how you are going to view the legal arguments."

The judges ruled against us. Their ruling was narrower than Judge Tingling's—it offered no talk about the Board of Health having author- ity only over "communicable, infectious, and pestilent diseases"—but it was nearly as bad. The Board of Health, they decided, was just another administrative agency. And then they decided that the *Boreali* criteria invalidated the rule. The rule must be solely about health, and the judges stretched to show that this rule wasn't. For example, I had commented at a board meeting that the rule might reduce obesity-related medical costs; the judges counted that as the board straying from health into economic considerations. The exceptions for fruit juice and milk-based beverages, and the fact that the rule did not apply to grocery stores, were not, in their view, health-based but instead "a compromise of social and economic concerns, as well as private interests."

As a sort of consolation prize, the judges wrote that "nothing in this decision is intended to circumscribe [the health department's] legitimate powers. Nor is this decision intended to express an opinion on the wisdom of the soda consumption restriction.... Within the limits described above, health authorities may make rules and regulations for the protection of public health."

To us in the health department, it wasn't much consolation. If these judges' ruling were to stand, the Board of Health still could not have passed crucial rules like the ban on lead paint, which had probably saved tens of thousands of children from lead poisoning. According to the judges, the board could act only as an administrative agency, under the instructions of the City Council.

We had one more shot, in the state's highest court. I asked the city's lawyers what they thought our chances were of winning there. Better than fifty-fifty, they said. I didn't believe them.

19

"It keeps me up at night."

It was in the tiny kitchen of Lucky's Café, just before Mayor Bloomberg's defiant press conference on the soda portion cap, that we started down a new track on smoking. Jim Gennaro, a talkative council member from Queens whose mother had died of lung cancer, had come to show his support for the portion rule. He collared me by the walk-in refrigerator. What did I think, he asked, about raising the legal sales age for cigarettes from eighteen to nineteen? Four states, including New Jersey, had already done it, as had neighboring Nassau and Suffolk Counties.

Gennaro was floating this proposal at a critical moment for our own antismoking ideas. It had been eight months since Mayor Bloomberg had agreed to prohibit the display of cigarette packs and to ban discount coupons for cigarettes. The next step for these two ideas would be to get backing from Speaker Christine Quinn, but between Hurricane Sandy and other issues with the City Council, it had taken months just to get the ideas in front of her. As 2013 began, with the mayor's race just a few months away, I was starting to lose hope.

To my amazement, when Speaker Quinn finally heard the ideas, she liked both. Long afterward I asked her why she was willing to push the bills against the opposition of the bodegas when she had so much at risk in the mayor's race. "Yeah, the bodega people are against you," she told me later, but that didn't bother her. "One, there were some things I just wasn't going to let politics be a part of. . . . And then two, just to make me not sound like a saint . . . people hate smoking. If you overlay primary voters with smoking, it's not really that controversial." She was running for mayor as The Candidate Who Gets Things Done. These were ideas that she wanted to claim.

In March 2013, when we were in the kitchen of Lucky's Café, we were preparing to unveil these two first-in-the-nation antismoking bills. When Gennaro told me his age-nineteen idea, my first reaction was that I just didn't want it to screw the two bills up.

A week later Mayor Bloomberg held a press conference at Queens Hospital to showcase our two bills. Several people buttressed him, including Matt Myers, the executive director for the national antismoking advocacy group Campaign for Tobacco-Free Kids, and Jim Gennaro. While the mayor gave equal time to the two bills, the reporters chose to focus on the one that hid cigarette packs. "We know out of sight doesn't always mean out of mind, but in many cases, it can," said Bloomberg. "We think this will help reduce impulse purchases, and if it does, it will literally save lives."

The tobacco companies were primed for this fight. A year earlier, the small town of Haverstraw, New York, had passed a tobacco product display ban; the corporations had quickly hit them with a lawsuit, brandishing the First Amendment's guarantee of free speech. Facing an army of tobacco lawyers, the town immediately folded, repealing the law. In their press statements, the tobacco companies now hinted that they would come after us in the same way. The bodega owners chimed in. "Where will it end?" said Bodega Association of the United States head Ramon Murphy. "Today it is cigarettes. Tomorrow it's soda. The next day it's chips. The following day it's sugar, and then ice cream. Before you know it, there are no bodegas left."

After Gennaro made his suggestion, Susan Kansagra looked into raising the tobacco sales age to nineteen and came back lukewarm. The one-year increase would do little to cut smoking in eighteen-year-olds or younger teens, because many would get their nineteen-year-old friends to buy cigarettes for them. We had invested years in our other two tobacco bills. Those had to come first.

Then Howard Wolfson called to ask what I thought about raising the legal sales age to twenty-one. Now Speaker Quinn's staff was asking. Age twenty-one was a very different question. Anyone over twenty-one was out of high school and was less likely to mingle with teens eighteen or younger. A study had found that 90 percent of people asked by teens to buy them cigarettes were under twenty-one. No states or big cities in the United States had raised their sales age to twenty-one, but a group of researchers had estimated that the law could immediately cut smoking rates in kids between fourteen and seventeen by two-thirds, and over fifty years cut smoking in adults by 30 percent.

We had a precedent arguing for the idea: when states raised the sales age for alcohol from eighteen to twenty-one, they saw big declines in drinking among high school seniors. A sales age of twenty-one would bring cigarettes in line with booze, making it easier to enforce the sale age of both. Later Vicki Grimshaw uncovered a statistical gem. In 2005 the small town of Needham, Massachusetts, had raised its tobacco sales age to twenty-one. From 2006 to 2012, smoking rates among Needham's high school students plummeted from 12.9 to 5.5 percent, a faster drop and to a lower point than had happened either in neighboring Massachusetts towns or in New York City. Seeing that, we told Quinn's staff that we wholeheartedly supported the idea.

In April 2013, Jim Gennaro and Christine Quinn came out with their age-twenty-one sales proposal. Reporters tracking the mayoral race saw political maneuvering. The *Times* reported that "by proposing the legislation, Ms. Quinn . . . appeared to be positioning herself to follow in [Bloomberg's] footsteps as a mayor who would make public health a priority." Quinn made it clear that she was jumping in with both feet. Soon afterward she persuaded state legislators in New Jersey, New York State, and Connecticut to introduce their own age-twenty-one bills.

. . .

In early May, the elegant City Council chambers were under renovation, so the health committee held its hearing in a drab office building across the street from City Hall. The committee would listen to testimony about three tobacco bills: the ban on displaying cigarette packs, the ban on discounting, and the age-twenty-one sales rule. As the hearing began, Christine Quinn dropped by to let the other council members know exactly where she stood. "There are few opportunities you have in life or in government to do something that you literally know will save lives," she said. "That is what we are talking about today."

Supporters and opponents overflowed the cramped room, lining the hallway. On the health side, organized by Susan Kansagra's team, were the usual antismoking advocacy organizations, the CEO of Memorial Sloan Kettering Cancer Center, professors who studied tobacco marketing, Marie (the star of our antismoking subway ads), and a representative of Price Chopper, a grocery chain that had voluntarily hidden its cigarette packs. On the other side was the retail end of the tobacco industry: grocery stores, bodegas, gas stations, and newsstands. Hiding the packs, of course, would damage an industry and kill jobs. "This is a joke," said David Schwartz of the New York Association of Grocery Stores. "This is an attack on small business. This is an assault on our grocery stores." Even though they were selling a killer drug, they presented themselves as upstanding community members. "There are millions of illegal cartons of cigarettes being sold in New York every day, and they are not being sold in stores," said Robert Bookman of the NYC Newsstand Operators Association. "They are being sold on the street. They are being sold from shopping bags. . . . They are being sold from trunks of cars. These bills do nothing to attack the tsunami of illegal cigarettes out there."

None of that surprised us. But just before the hearing, I was puzzled to see a small cluster of people carrying handwritten posters about "vaping." What's that about? I asked Kevin Schroth. They're advocates for electronic cigarettes, he said, upset because in drafting the bills, he had changed the definition of "tobacco product." A possible unintended effect of that, which he hadn't recognized until just before the hearing, was that the bill would ban the sale of flavored e-cigarettes.

After my testimony, one of the first questions the health committee chair asked me was what effect the bills would have on e-cigarettes. I was still confused. "The bills were written with no intention of addressing electronic cigarettes at all," I said, hesitating. "If that is a concern of the council, I think that that is something that we can address in a subsequent conversation." Still, the e-cigarette advocates were determined to defend them. As the hearing, which started at 1:30 p.m., dragged on into the evening hours, a parade of "vapers" came to the witness table to implore the few remaining council members. "I quit smoking after eighteen years from an electronic cigarette," said Keith Mortener. "It saved my life I feel. It saved my mother's life and many people I know."

With Quinn's strong-arming, the few City Council members who sat through the hearing made the right noises about our three bills. After years of planning and months of preparation, we sensed victory. But the questions about e-cigarettes, which we saw as a minor glitch, later put them all at risk.

• • •

The epidemiologists were—only half-jokingly—calling it the *"Mad Men* effect." I was calling it a disaster. Even a year later, Susan Kansagra told me, "It keeps me up at night."

In the summer of 2013 we got the results of the 2012 telephone survey, and the smoking rate was 15.5 percent. That was up from 14.8 percent the year before, which was itself above the 14.0 percent in 2010 that Mayor Bloomberg had announced in his victory press conference. The 2012 number translated to an increase of 100,000 smokers in those two years.

The rising numbers could have been random noise in the surveys. But they followed eight years of consistent falls that amounted to 450,000 fewer smokers. Any increase after that represented a tragic reversal. At best, the quitters in New York City were matched by those picking up the deadly habit, and at worst, they were swamped by a surge of new smokers.

More than the increase itself, what struck the epidemiologists were the demographics of the new smokers. The greatest rises were among whites, males, those ages twenty-four to forty-four, those with a college education, and those in the highest income group. That was another radical change, because over the decades smoking had previously shifted to poor, less-educated people.

I was as distraught as I had been during my entire time on the job. Both Tom Frieden and I had called smoking public health enemy number one. The annual drops in smoking for nearly a decade had been the health department's greatest achievement. We had kept up the effort. What could be going wrong?

Some answers were right in front of us. The cigarette taxes were stale; after a price shock prompts many smokers to quit, others adjust. The tobacco companies were stringing some smokers along with discount coupons, and the cigarette smugglers trucking in cartons from Virginia were holding down the actual retail price. City budget cuts that followed the financial crash of 2008 had also hurt us: in 2006 we had spent over $8 million on antismoking ads, but between 2010 and 2012 we had cut back to $5.5 million a year. Over the same time, the state health department had sliced its own antismoking ad buys roughly in half for the same reason. With fewer ads on television, the number of people calling the Quitline was down from about 150,000 to about 100,000 a year.

But something else was happening. New Yorkers were changing the way they smoked. In 1980 the average smoker went through a pack and a half a day; now nearly 40 percent of smokers in New York City didn't light a single cigarette on any given day. These "nondailies" didn't even consider themselves smokers.

The wildly successful television series *Mad Men*, which began in 2007, was billed by AMC as a "sexy, stylized, and provocative" drama that "follows the lives of the ruthlessly competitive men and women of Madison Avenue advertising" in the 1960s. Throughout nearly every scene, the hyperaggressive men—almost all of whom are white, educated, wealthy, and attractive—smoke.

Watching actors smoke in movies, the surgeon general has said, causes

young people to start smoking. That conclusion came from various studies. In one of the best, researchers repeatedly surveyed more than 2,000
children aged nine to twelve, who had never before experimented with
smoking, about the movies they had seen. The researchers then watched
those movies and counted the scenes in which the actors smoked. Over
five years, the more smoking scenes the children watched, the more likely
they were to try cigarettes, even after taking into account whether their
parents or friends smoked. The researchers projected that the number of
children trying cigarettes would fall by one-third if none of them watched
smoking on screen.

The invention of on-demand television now had Americans watching
series like *Mad Men*—which was effectively a steady stream of cigarette
ads—instead of broadcast cop dramas. I suspected, but couldn't prove,
that those series were giving New Yorkers a much heavier dose of alluring smoking images. Maybe those images were causing higher-income,
educated people to take up "social smoking."

Smoking a few cigarettes a week isn't nearly as dangerous as smoking
a pack a day, but it can still be fatal. Shows like *Mad Men* might not have
been the only factor behind the distressing survey numbers. But it was
painfully clear that in response to our antismoking program, the tobacco
companies were adapting somehow. The war against the cigarette sellers
would never end. We needed to rethink our strategy quickly, as they had
rethought theirs. If we didn't, smoking could come roaring back.

At the health department, we couldn't rewrite television shows. Susan
Kansagra came up with a plan for what we actually could do. We should
find the money to counter the *Mad Men*–like images with antismoking
ads, ones that resonated with light smokers and nondaily smokers. We
should crack down on bodegas that sold cheap bootleg cigarettes. And we
absolutely had to get the City Council to pass the three bills restricting
cigarette marketing in retail stores.

. . .

As the summer of 2013 dragged on, though, and the election approached,
Christine Quinn's office repeatedly delayed the vote on the three bills.

During those delays, the bills came under threat not from politicians but from the antismoking advocates.

Under Quinn's iron hand, the City Council had looked favorably on all three. We wanted only to nail down the victories. But after the American Heart Association, the American Lung Association, the American Cancer Society, and the Campaign for Tobacco-Free Kids learned at the hearing that the bills might inadvertently restrict electronic cigarettes, they perked up and decided that the bills should do just that.

Kevin Schroth guessed that the antismoking groups were panicked by recent announcements by both R.J. Reynolds and Philip Morris that they were jumping into the e-cigarette business. Soon all three big tobacco companies would be marketing e-cigarettes heavily. Everything the tobacco corporations did had to be countered, the advocates' reasoning went, so if the tobacco companies were putting billions behind e-cigarettes, then health people had to do whatever it took to thwart them.

Electronic cigarettes are devices that deliver nicotine, the drug in tobacco leaves to which smokers get addicted. They contain a cartridge filled with a liquid like propylene glycol, in which nicotine is dissolved. When a user sucks on an e-cigarette, a microprocessor heats the liquid, which sends out a puff of vapor carrying the nicotine into the user's lungs. A pharmacist in China invented the device in 2003 and started exporting e-cigarettes a couple of years later. Soon U.S.-based entrepreneurs and investors with tech roots started up companies like NJOY and Blu to market their own versions. When those e-cigarettes started to catch on, the tobacco companies hedged their bets: Lorillard bought Blu for $135 million in 2012 before R.J. Reynolds and Philip Morris created their own brands in 2013.

In 2009 the FDA seized a shipment of NJOY's e-cigarettes from China to the United States, calling them unapproved drug-delivery devices. NJOY and other e-cigarette companies sued, arguing that since the nicotine in e-cigarettes was derived from tobacco, they were actually like cigarettes and therefore should instead fall under the FDA's much looser rules regulating tobacco products. In a mystifying decision, a federal judge agreed with them. His ruling left the FDA paralyzed in the short term and hampered by the federal tobacco laws in the long term. As of 2013, the FDA had done nothing to regulate the chemicals that companies put in e-cigarette cartridges. Neither the FDA nor any other federal agency prevented manufacturers from advertising e-cigarettes in any way, stores from selling them anywhere to anyone, or users from puffing on them anyplace. E-cigarettes sprouted in bodegas throughout New York City, including those without tobacco licenses.

The manufacturers advertised them in magazines, on billboards, and on television, using the tactics that cigarette manufacturers had used to advertise Kool and Marlboro forty years earlier, with celebrities and with images linking them to youth, independence, rebelliousness, and sex. In one ad, punk rocker Courtney Love, puffing at an elegant event, is approached by an older woman who tells her haughtily that she "can't smoke in here." Love blows vapor in the woman's face and says with a sneer, "Relax. It's a fuckin' NJOY." Blu ran an ad in the *Sports Illustrated* swimsuit edition with its logo applied right over the crotch of a model's tiny bikini, with the slogan "Slim. Charged. Ready to go." By 2012, the companies were selling $500 million worth of e-cigarettes. Wall Street analysts were predicting that sales would double in 2013 and might surpass those of tobacco cigarettes within a decade.

The e-cigarette companies profited from having it both ways. Because the FDA couldn't regulate e-cigarettes as drugs, the companies could market them with everything from free giveaways to sales at gas stations. At the same time, although the companies couldn't claim that e-cigarettes helped smokers quit, they could drop loud hints. "Cigarettes, you've met your match," says one NJOY ad. The companies recruited vapers to say the devices helped them quit and to fight any attempt to regulate e-cigarettes; government interference, they said, would simply force them back to "combustion" cigarettes and early death.

Some legitimate public health experts thought e-cigarettes had the potential to save many lives by replacing smoking. Propylene glycol is harmless, they argued, used in many inhalers licensed by the FDA, and nicotine by itself is a safe drug—the active ingredient in the patches and gum that the health department distributes to help smokers quit. The patches and gums didn't work for most smokers; something that delivered nicotine to the lungs in a way that felt like smoking might work better. If even a third of smokers were to switch from inhaling tobacco smoke to sucking on e-cigarettes, it might save tens of thousands of lives a year.

In 2013 e-cigarettes were still so new that public health officials couldn't answer the crucial questions about their health risks. What were their long-term effects? The FDA called propylene glycol safe, but no one had ever heated it up and then breathed in the vapor for hours every day for twenty years. If young people got addicted to nicotine through e-cigarettes, would some then switch to tobacco? Would smokers use e-cigarettes not as a way to quit but as a way to *avoid* quitting—a "bridge" that would just tide them over during the workday? (Blu played on that, with ad copy that said, "Why Quit? Switch to Blu.")

At the health department, we staked our reputation on following scientific evidence. Without studies on e-cigarettes, we had difficulty arguing to regulate them. But with the market exploding, City Hall would soon be crawling with e-cigarette lobbyists. Then it might be too late.

We needed to balance the possible benefits of e-cigarettes with the risks of their unfettered marketing. The closest analogy was methadone, which health agencies recommend for heroin addicts under the label "harm reduction." Methadone is a risky and addictive drug, but it is far safer than heroin. Heroin addicts who switch to daily methadone can lead healthy, productive lives for years. But we recommend methadone only to people who are already addicted. We would never allow sales of methadone to teenagers in bodegas or the advertising of methadone on television. If e-cigarettes ever became the "harm reduction" for tobacco, they should still never be marketed to nonsmokers. But the e-cigarette manufacturers were flagrantly marketing the devices to nonsmokers, because there were so many more of them.

It made sense to include e-cigarettes in the age-twenty-one sales law. Few under-twenty-ones were fully addicted smokers, so they shouldn't need the e-cigarettes to quit, but all of them could be easily lured into trying e-cigarettes and becoming addicted to nicotine. I couldn't justify, though, including e-cigarettes in the pack display ban or the discount ban. How would we argue—in public, in the City Council, or in court—that this would be good for health when there were no data showing that e-cigarettes were bad?

The antitobacco advocates, though, wanted to define e-cigarettes as cigarettes, which would mean that all three of the bills would apply. If we didn't include e-cigarettes in the pack display ban, they told us, stores would just replace the cigarette-pack power walls with displays for e-cigarettes. As time passed, the advocates only became more insistent. By the end of the summer, the American Heart Association, the American Lung Association, and the American Cancer Society lobbyists stunned us by saying they would now refuse to support the three bills *unless* they applied to e-cigarettes.

In the middle of that argument, the director for the Campaign for Tobacco-Free Kids inserted an entirely different demand. He believed that, because federal judges were now so expansive in interpreting protected commercial speech, the bill requiring retailers to hide cigarette packs would lose a lawsuit by the tobacco companies. And a federal court ruling like that, if it were broad, might hurt other antismoking policies, like the FDA's rule requiring that cigarette packs carry pictorial warnings. He didn't want New York City to pass the pack display ban, with or without e-cigarettes. The pressure of the powerful tobacco companies had split even those of us who agreed that tobacco was the nation's top public enemy.

These groups mattered because Christine Quinn felt she needed all the antismoking groups standing with her. As she explained later, the bills were confusing, they were "pushing the envelope," and they weren't the council's idea. How could she force the bills through the chamber if even the antismoking people wouldn't support them? She called the lobbyist for Tobacco-Free Kids and "had a firm conversation with him" in which she threatened to "walk away from everything," but he didn't budge. "I couldn't believe it," said Quinn. "It was just so insane!"

Hoping to get help out of the morass, I went to Mayor Bloomberg. As we sat at a table in the Bull Pen, I told him that three of the four antismoking groups were insisting that we include e-cigarettes in the tobacco bills and that the fourth wanted to kill the pack display ban because of legal risks. I want to pass all of them without changes, I said, hoping that he could persuade Quinn. If the council were to pass these groundbreaking bills, I believed the advocates would fall in line.

The Bloomberg administration had just been stung by court losses over the sugary drink portion cap and a requirement that taxicabs be gasoline-electric hybrids. We saw these defeats as inevitable turf battles among different arms of a checks-and-balances government, but the public, Howard Wolfson said, saw them as the mayor breaking the law. We couldn't afford another loss in court, he thought.

Bloomberg listened. If there's a real risk that we'll lose the pack display ban in court, he said, pull it back.

That left us with the age-twenty-one bill and the bill that would ban price discounts. We agreed to include e-cigarettes in the age-twenty-one bill. Then we persuaded the antismoking advocates that there was no practical way to prohibit discounting of e-cigarettes when the product was not standardized. And we went back to Christine Quinn with an agreement on the two bills.

In September 2013, Quinn's long campaign for mayor ended. She had been first in the polls for months but saw her lead disintegrate in the month before the primary, not just to second, which would have given her a chance in a runoff against a surging Bill de Blasio, but to third. Afterward, she was no longer a candidate but still speaker, so she went back to doing what she did best: passing bills. She brought the two antismoking bills up for votes. Few council members spoke in opposition to either, but those who did complained about the age-twenty-one sales restriction. If someone is old enough to go to war, they argued, he should be old enough to buy cigarettes. But as Vicki Grimshaw put it, "I don't understand why if you can die for your country, you can die for the tobacco industry. I don't get that parallel." The age-twenty-one sales limit passed by a vote of 35 to 10. The bill that banned discounts on cigarettes, set a minimum price, required "bundling" of cigars, and gave the city, in the words of the Bloomberg press release, "new tools to crack down on disreputable retailers and black-market bootleggers," passed by an even larger margin of 36 to 9.

The antismoking advocates and the health department put aside the painful arguments over the now-dead pack display ban and went to a (smoke-free) bar near City Hall to celebrate the success not just of these two bills but of the Bloomberg administration's twelve years of work against tobacco. "It was great," said Grimshaw. And then "it was like, Okay, how long will it take before the industry serves us with a lawsuit?"

. . .

We thought that would be the last word on tobacco. It wasn't. Council member Jim Gennaro called us after the vote to say he wanted to "ban e-cigarettes." By that he meant to include them the Smoke-Free Air Act, which would prohibit using e-cigarettes in restaurants, bars, and other workplaces.

Despite her waning days as speaker—or maybe because of them—Christine Quinn was game. "Two things happened," she explained to me. "One, it was like, what the fuck, let's give it a shot. You know what I mean. Let's go out with a bang." And then "I wanted to allow members the ability to say 'You know what, I didn't leave not having gotten X passed.'" And she hated e-cigarettes. "Whether the data show it or not, younger people are going to get them, and it's going to put you on a life of smoking," she told me. "You don't have to be a scientist or doctor to know that. It's common sense. . . . And there's nicotine in them! . . . So this is *not good*! This is *bad*!"

Mayor Bloomberg, when we spoke about it, reacted even more strongly. "They're just trying to get young people hooked," he said, disgusted.

I saw other reasons for banning e-cigarettes indoors. Later I phrased it this way: Imagine a crowded bar filled with people puffing on things that look like cigarettes. If a bartender then smells tobacco smoke, whom would he tap on the shoulder and ask to put the cigarette out? If we allowed e-cigarettes in bars, the Smoke-Free Air Act itself, which depended on enforcement by employees and bystanders, might unravel. And if conventional cigarettes crept back into bars, we would lose Bloomberg's society-altering achievement of 2002, which was one of the best things anyone had done in the history of smoking prevention.

By the time of the hearing on the e-cigarette bill, the renovations had been completed in City Hall, and we were back in the council's grand chamber. The majestic room was outfitted with dark wood wainscoting, mahogany desks, deep red carpeting, and life-size portraits of the Marquis de Lafayette and of George Washington beside a white horse. That day dozens of e-cigarette vapers packed the gallery to listen and be heard. Throughout the four-and-a-half-hour hearing, as they murmured and applauded and heckled, they also sucked and puffed on various e-cigarette contraptions, sending out plumes of fruity vapor. And that made our case for us.

Council member Peter Vallone told the crowd, "I'm watching puffs of vapor go up in this room, and it is confusing, number one. And number two, I smell it. It doesn't bother me. It smells good. But it might bother me if I were in a restaurant and I smelled that." One of our legislative staff members on the scene found it hilarious. "It smelled almost like bad room deodorizer," she said. "It was like, what *not* to do if you want to convince electeds of something."

Several e-cigarette advocates even puffed away as they testified. "All the Council members were offended," said another health department employee. Christine Quinn said later, "What a group of freaks! Who the hell knew there was going to be this pack of weirdos who showed up and smoked e-cigarettes in the chambers! Bizarre!"

When the council met two weeks later on December 19, on their last meeting before the new administration took over and before many members were forced out by term limits, the body voted to include electronic cigarettes in the Smoke-Free Air Act by a tally of 43 to 8.

. . .

And there was one last twist before the bill would become law, a coda to the Bloomberg administration's long war on smoking.

On December 26, 2013, five days before Mike Bloomberg ended his twelve-year run as mayor of New York City, he and I met with Sean Parker, the brash tech entrepreneur who cofounded Napster and had been the first president of Facebook. At thirty-four, Parker had already founded or invested in many start-ups, been chased from three companies, and accumulated $2 billion. Another tech entrepreneur called him "the Picasso of business," but a profile in *Forbes* had described him as "flighty, manic and unpredictable." Parker had invested tens of millions in NJOY, the e-cigarette company that proclaims, "Our mission is to obsolete cigarettes." Wearing jeans and a trim, reddish-brown beard, he arrived in Bloomberg's Bull Pen to persuade the mayor to veto the bill including e-cigarettes in the Smoke-Free Air Act.

After making small talk with Bloomberg about where they were investing their billions and the foolishly high stock price of Twitter, Parker began to make his case. Before he got rolling, though, the mayor told him calmly that "we're too far into this" to back out now.

Parker went on anyway. He wasn't investing in e-cigarettes to make money. He was only in NJOY to make people healthier. The tobacco industry was a typical, traditional, "fucked-up market." Government regulation of tobacco hadn't achieved much and—as always when government tried to interfere with markets—was bound to fail. But e-cigarettes were going to disrupt that market. They were already winning market share from combustion cigarettes, and they were still in version 1.0. Future versions were bound to outcompete Marlboro. When they did, they would do more to end smoking and promote health than anything government would ever do. Given their potential, Bloomberg shouldn't do anything to interfere with e-cigarettes, especially prohibit people from using them indoors.

The mayor looked bored and distracted and mostly left it up to me to respond. It would be one thing if NJOY were trying to help smokers quit, I jumped in. If NJOY wanted to end smoking, the company should do the studies that showed that e-cigarettes were safe and effective for quitting and then get licensed by the FDA for that. If NJOY did that, public health people like me would be the company's loudest cheerleaders. But NJOY was behaving like a pure for-profit company, and the profit in e-cigarettes was in getting nonsmokers addicted. The company's marketing—like sending hunky bare-chested men to pass out free samples in Union Square—seemed to be all about capturing young nonsmokers.

Parker wasn't impressed. It dawned on me that he and I saw the world entirely differently. He believed in the limitless potential of technological innovation and free markets to make the world better. I believed government needed to protect citizens from profit-driven corporations selling products that hurt people. We weren't going to agree.

The more Parker pressed his case, the more distracted Bloomberg looked. The mayor glanced around the Bull Pen and commented on other things he was working on. But he came back to e-cigarettes just enough to confirm, calmly, that he couldn't possibly veto a bill that his administration had pushed.

With just five days left, Parker shot back, Bloomberg could do whatever he wanted.

Bloomberg's attention was wandering further afield, so the conversation became one between Parker and me. He became increasingly agitated as he kept arguing, as if he were a kettle about to boil. Eventually the mayor, looking more bored than ever, stood up and walked back into the sea of desks. And then Parker left, red-faced.

• • •

On December 30, 2013, with less than forty-eight hours left in his mayoralty, Mike Bloomberg held a bill-signing ceremony in the Blue Room, the last of hundreds. Christine Quinn's last-minute flurry of legislating had given him twenty-two to sign. It was a bookend of sorts. One of his earliest bills had banned smoking in bars and restaurants. One of the last would prohibit using a high-tech cigarette substitute in the same places.

The Blue Room was packed with reporters and curious onlookers. Jim Gennaro was there, proud of himself and full of praise for the mayor. Bloomberg, standing behind the podium with the mayoral seal and beside the portrait of Alexander Hamilton, was a touch nostalgic. When he opened up the floor for comments, several doctors and health advocates who had traveled to City Hall for the moment came to the mike to extol not just the e-cigarette bill but Bloomberg's dozen years protecting New Yorkers' health. They were followed by two angry smokers who, with comments like "good people disobey bad laws," lit up cigarettes in front of the news cameras. "Okay," Bloomberg said to them calmly, "I think it's time to leave."

20

"That is, ultimately, government's highest duty."

On September 20, 2011, I entered the General Assembly Hall at the United Nations with a small group of city officials. The UN was holding a high-level meeting to "launch an all-out attack on non-communicable diseases (NCDs)"—including heart disease, stroke, cancer, diabetes, and chronic lung disease—"the often preventable scourge that causes 63 per cent of all deaths." It was only the second such meeting in the organization's history on a health topic; the other had been held ten years earlier on HIV/AIDS. The General Assembly Hall is an oval cavern trimmed in green and gold. The ceiling was lost several stories above us, and the floor below was filled with desks bearing labels like Paraguay and Estonia. Balcony seats ring three-quarters of the oval, and behind them are glass-windowed booths for interpreters. At the front, beneath a giant wooden backdrop holding the UN logo, is a green-marbled desk for the UN leaders, in front of which stands a speaker's lectern.

It was my first time at the UN. Although I had been warned, I found it even more chaotic than advertised. When we arrived, speaking behind the lectern was the president of Hungary, who was followed by the prime minister of St. Kitts and Nevis. As the heads of state spoke, delegates at their tables chatted with one another, tapped on their cell phones, or milled around. But when these speakers finished and the next one rose to

256 Tom Farley, MD

the podium, the delegates sat up, lifted their cell phones, and began snapping pictures, their flashes flickering across the floor. They were seeing
New York City's mayor, Michael Bloomberg.

For more than 150 years, most governments had assumed that the only
diseases worth preventing were caused by infections that passed from one
person to another. And even in 2012, the communicable diseases of HIV,
tuberculosis, and malaria persisted. But as the twentieth century became
the twenty-first, the diseases that killed most humans had changed dras-
tically. With sanitation, vaccination, and nutrition subduing infectious
diseases, NCDs had come to the fore. This "epidemiologic transition"
hit countries at different times, but the change reached every corner of
the world. In the United States, fewer than 5 percent of deaths were from
communicable diseases, and 88 percent were from NCDs. Between 1990
and 2010, Mexico had begun to look like the United States, as deaths
from communicable diseases dropped from 19 to 7 percent and those
from NCDs rose from 56 to 77 percent. India of 2010 looked like Mexico
of 1990 and was changing quickly. It seems inevitable that sub-Saharan
Africa, the last holdout for the scourge of infectious diseases, will follow
India within the life spans of most people living there today. Globally, for
every person killed by natural disasters in 2010, NCDs killed 175 people.
For every one killed by war, NCDs killed 1,950.

NCDs aren't just signs of old age. In fact, many of them are easy to
prevent. "Knowing how to reduce such diseases is not the problem," a
report of the secretary-general read. "The problem is lack of action." The
report went on, "The greatest reductions in non-communicable diseases
will come from population-wide interventions to address the risk factors
of tobacco use, unhealthy diet, lack of physical activity, and harmful use
of alcohol." Mike Bloomberg was now at the podium to tell the world's
leaders how he had done that.

*Improving public health has long been one of my passions, and it's why
I'm devoted to enhancing one of the world's preeminent schools of public
health at my alma mater, the Johns Hopkins University, which is dedicated to saving lives, millions at a time.*

In the early 1990s, according to Al Sommer, "public health was a backwater." Even the term felt outdated and distasteful; to many, public health meant "washing your hands, flushing the toilet, and poor docs for poor people." But with his donation to Johns Hopkins, Bloomberg had made public health "a legitimate enterprise, gotten students excited about doing it, gotten donors excited about investing in it, and created a global movement." Between 2000 and 2014, graduate schools of public health in the United States more than doubled in number, from 28 to 60. Other schools of public health acquired the names of new-economy philanthropists, from Michael Milken at George Washington University to T. H. Chan at Harvard. And Johns Hopkins and other leading universities had established undergraduate programs in public health that students flocked to.

We have made reducing noncommunicable disease the focus of public health policy here in New York City, a city of about 8.4 million people. And I'm happy to report that we have had considerable success as a result. It's fundamental to why for New Yorkers today, life expectancy has increased faster and remains higher than for Americans overall.

Mike Bloomberg often quipped, "If you want your friends and relatives to live long, healthy lives, tell them to move to New York City." His audience usually laughed, but it wasn't a joke. Between 2001 and 2010, life expectancy at birth in New York City increased 3.0 years to 80.9 years. In the United States as a whole during that decade, life expectancy rose only 1.8 years, to 78.7. For most of the twentieth century, New York City residents had had a shorter life expectancy than other Americans. The gap the city opened up in 2010 was the largest in history. The renaissance in health wasn't just an urban trend, because New York City had a faster rise in life expectancy in the twenty-first century than every other major city in the United States

By the time Mike Bloomberg was finishing his third term, articles were appearing in scientific journals trying to explain New York City's increasing life expectancy. One theory credited New York's strong economy, poverty being linked to disease and earlier death. But life expectancy had climbed even while New York City's poverty rate barely budged. A pair of demographers attributed the longer life expectancy in 2010 to immigration, because New York has many newcomers, and immigrants traditionally are healthier than people born in the United States. But from 2000 to 2010, as life expectancy in the city surged, the proportion of New Yorkers born abroad did not change, and it was actually U.S.-born New Yorkers whose life expectancy grew faster than that of Americans elsewhere.

Of the city's increase in life expectancy during this decade, 50 percent was due to declines in heart disease and 16 percent to falls in cancer, the causes of death that Tom Frieden had decided to attack in 2002. Those were also the two disease categories most directly linked to smoking. From 2000 until 2012, the number of New Yorkers who died annually of ischemic heart disease (the type caused by smoking, unhealthy diet, and physical inactivity) dropped by more than 8,000. Tom Frieden would count those as lives saved.

No one can be certain what caused New Yorkers' life expectancy to grow so quickly during the Bloomberg years. Most of the years of healthy life that city residents will enjoy from lower smoking rates, healthier diets, and more physical activity will show up far in the future. The long life of New Yorkers today, though, is a hopeful sign of even more gains to come.

At the outset of our administration, we recognized that noncommunicable diseases—especially heart disease and cancer—far outstripped all other causes of death in our city and that the single most effective thing that we could do to reduce them was to discourage smoking.

In New York City in 2014, people did not smoke in restaurants. They did not smoke in bars. They could not smoke on hospital grounds. Far fewer than before smoked in parks and on beaches. In bodegas, cigarettes costs about $11 per pack. On television and in subways, ads reminded children and adults of the suffering that comes from smoking. And a dozen years after Tom Frieden demanded that doctors offer treatment to their smoking patients, the health department was assisting more than half the city's doctors do that. Those doctors were asking about 8 in 10 patients about smoking and counseling half their smoking patients to quit.

In the later Bloomberg years, the city became a proving ground for new ideas to fight smoking. Some, like the mandated warning signs and the ban on pack displays in stores, didn't survive legal or political battles, but they remain ready for others to try. Others, like raising the age of cigarette sales to twenty-one and ending discount coupons, became law.

Three months after the City Council passed the discount ban, the National Association of Tobacco Outlets sued, attempting to detonate both nuclear weapons. It argued that the law was preempted because it interfered with cigarette "promotion and advertising," and that it violated tobacco companies' First Amendment right to free speech by blocking their ability to tell customers that they were "getting a deal." This time the city won. In 2014 the coupons and the "$2 off!" signs disappeared from bodegas. Appearing in their place were signs demanding that cigarette customers prove they were over twenty-one.

The Bloomberg administration's antismoking policies worked. Between 2002 and 2011, smoking among adult New Yorkers fell by 31 percent, compared to 16 percent among all Americans. Smoking rates among New York's high school students fell 52 percent—compared to 36 percent in the United States as a whole—to a rate that was less than half the national rate. But the tobacco industry adapted, using every legal technique of marketing to push sales back up. Racks of shiny cigarette packs and eye-catching cigarette ads stood behind the cash registers at Walgreens. While little cigarette-like cigars now sold for at least $10.50 a pack because of the new city law, slightly larger cigarillos appeared in bodegas selling in four-packs for 99 cents. Onscreen smoking by movie actors stayed high, and smoking filled many television shows. Meanwhile, e-cigarettes were beginning to look like a fad, as national sales in 2014 leveled and market researchers said that regular smokers, after experimenting, were going back to the real thing.

In New York City, the rebound in smoking continued into 2013—rising by 0.6 percent to 16.1 percent—as did the downshift toward nondaily smoking. In 2014 the health department's newest ad campaign slogan tried to speak directly to nondaily smokers with taglines like "cancer doesn't care you 'don't smoke that much.'"

> *By the end of the decade, the WHO [World Health Organization] expects 7.5 million tobacco-related deaths worldwide, every year. Some 80 percent of these deaths will take place in the world's low- and middle-income nations—nations where tobacco companies have stepped up their marketing briskly. . . . That's why I've also made tobacco control a major priority of Bloomberg Philanthropies.*

By 2014, two-thirds of the U.S. population lived in places with smoke-free restaurants and bars, and most of Europe was covered by smoke-free air laws. The Bloomberg money took the New York City program to the rest of the world. Between 2007 and 2012, Bloomberg Philanthropies spent $375 million to train government officials, advocates, reporters, and lawyers in dozens of poorer countries in the MPOWER strategy. In 2012, Kelly Henning traveled to Bangladesh, a country of over 150 million in which nearly half of men smoked, to meet with its health minister. A year before, the foundation had paid for the health minister's assistant to come to the United States for training. On the wall of the room where the assistant worked—the only thing on the wall—was a picture of him receiving his course certificate. That assistant was crucial to Bangladesh's passing a law that required graphic warnings on cigarette packs and that banned smoking in many indoor places.

Between 2007 and 2012, twenty-six low- and middle-income countries passed comprehensive smoke-free air laws. That quadrupled the number of people worldwide protected from secondhand smoke to 1.1 billion, or 16 percent of the world's population. In 2014, in what may become the biggest win, Beijing passed a strong indoor smoking ban, and China published draft regulations for a national ban.

The Bloomberg foundation also paid for antismoking ad campaigns in poorer countries, often using ads from New York City. By 2012 more than half of the world's population lived in countries that were running national media campaigns against smoking. After Vietnam aired *Cigarettes*

Are Eating You Alive, a survey showed that most of the nation remembered seeing it, and more than three-quarters of the smokers who had seen it said the ad made them more likely to quit.

Turkey tried every element of MPOWER, banning smoking in restaurants and bars, banning tobacco retail ads, raising its cigarette tax to 80 percent of the retail price, and requiring television stations to run antitobacco programs in prime time. Within four years the country's smoking rate dropped from 32 to 27 percent, a fall of 1.2 million smokers.

A researcher from Georgetown, working with the Bloomberg foundation, estimated that the declines in smoking between 2007 and 2012 from use of the MPOWER strategy in sixty-five countries would prevent 14 million premature deaths.

The progress we're seeing on tobacco is encouraging action on other fronts as well. To attack diabetes and heart attacks, for example, in New York, we have also taken the lead in promoting healthier eating.

In 2013 a huge study on health risks around the world blamed unhealthy eating in America for 675,000 annual deaths, or one-fourth of all deaths. Americans consume way too much sodium, processed meat, trans fat, and sugar—especially from sugary drinks—and not nearly enough fruit, vegetables, nuts, seeds, whole grains, or fiber. Most of the biological havoc wreaked by unhealthy eating is invisible until people are stricken by heart disease, stroke, cancer, or diabetes, but the most visible harm—obesity—is frighteningly common.

When Frieden started, he drew on proven ideas to fight smoking, but he had no rulebook for promoting healthier eating across a city of eight million. Most public health experts were still focused on educating people, usually one at a time, to choose healthier food. Around that time, though, some experts like Mary Bassett and Lynn Silver saw the problem not as a lack of education but instead as a "toxic food environment." In the Bloomberg years, the New York City health department tried to detoxify that environment.

That meant banning trans fats in restaurants, requiring calorie labels on menu boards, licensing Green Carts, cutting salt in processed food, writing healthy food standards wherever the city had influence, and pushing policies to blunt the marketing of soda. Most of those ideas succeeded. No one in New York City is eating doughnuts soaked in trans fats, and none go to New Jersey to buy their French fries. The calorie labels on menu boards, while making only a small difference, seem to be having a greater impact as people get familiar with them. On a typical day, as Mike Bloomberg finished his term, about 250 Green Carts sold fresh produce on the sidewalks of the city's poorest neighborhoods. While the bodegas had protested that the competition would hurt them, it seems to have helped their customers; in neighborhoods where the Green Carts were active, the brick-and-mortar stores' offerings of fruits and vegetables actually increased. "I don't know, did their Cheetos sales go down?" asked Christine Quinn. "I hope so."

The city's food policy coordinator, working with the health department, quietly expanded the reach of the city's food standards. By 2013 the city had a single set of detailed health criteria for the food and beverages that were distributed by twelve city agencies or sold in more than 3,000 vending machines in government buildings. For the first time, the schools paid attention to how much sugar, sodium, and fiber were in the breakfast cereal they served. Some manufacturers altered junk food to barely meet the criteria—like creating reduced-sugar, whole-grain Pop-Tarts—but overall the foods were healthier. Deep-fried potato chips disappeared from vending machines, replaced by almonds and raisins. In 2010 the health department packaged a set of healthy food standards for hospitals, including rules for patient meals, vending machines, and cafeteria foods. By 2013, more than thirty of the city's fifty hospitals were following one or more standards.

In the fall of 2014, the health department was still working with twenty-three companies to cut salt in processed food. Christine Curtis thought the city's salt targets themselves—high enough to be feasible but low enough to matter—were an accomplishment, because before them the sky had been the limit. Food companies started checking the targets as they developed new recipes.

But the National Salt Reduction Initiative desperately needed the FDA in order to succeed, because only the FDA could set requirements for packaged food. Through 2014, we heard rumors that the FDA was poised to start a voluntary salt-reduction program, but that the White House was blocking the plan. By November 2014—more than three years after the FDA released its sodium docket, and more than six years after New York City's Salt Summit—the FDA still had done nothing on salt. Meanwhile other countries made headway; in 2013 the government of South Africa became the first to pass a sodium-reduction law with food standards that were mandatory.

In fact, the actions most needed to protect people from unhealthy food of all kinds had to come from the FDA and the other big federal food agency, the Department of Agriculture. Unfortunately, the USDA saw its mission as promoting agriculture, not health, and the FDA had been muzzled by a White House that listened far too much to the food companies. In late 2013 the FDA issued a "preliminary determination" on trans fats that might someday lead to a ban but a year later had not taken additional steps. The agency did finally act on menu calorie labeling in December 2014, shortly after the midterm election and nearly five years after Congress passed the law requiring it. Under the rules, not only restaurants but also grocery stores, bodegas, and convenience stores that sell prepared food—like 7-Elevens— would be required to post calorie labels. Those stores criticized the rules and persuaded friends in Congress to propose bills that would roll back the requirements.

The New York City health department spent more time on sugary drinks than on any other problem. In the last months of the Bloomberg administration, the department continued to run counter-ads on television and on subways, encouraged hundreds of community groups to rid themselves of sugary drinks, and extended a prohibition from day care centers to day camps.

As the term wound down, the sugary drink portion cap became a headache for Bloomberg. Other politicians ribbed him about it at events. The annual press satire of City Hall was entitled "Last Gulp." *The New Yorker* ran covers on it. The late-night comics couldn't resist coming back to it. Newspaper retrospectives listed it as an example of Bloomberg's tendency to overreach. Bloomberg, ever game, went with it: when Seth Meyers on *Saturday Night Live* asked him about his future, he said he would be "fulfilling a lifelong dream of enjoying a small soda on a nonsmoking beach." Through it all, he never once complained to me or to his deputy mayors about the spin.

In June 2014 six judges of New York State's highest court heard arguments over the portion cap. This last round of the case had become a magnet for advocates and legal experts. Coming to the city's side were professors of New York constitutional law, national public health advocates, and a group of New York City–based minority organizations. The last group wrote, "For the one of every three children born in 2000 who will develop type 2 diabetes, and for the one of every two African-American and Hispanic girls who will get the disease, the question is not whether the Rule was justified, but rather 'What else is being done?'" Joining the soda companies were thirty-two members of the City Council and the Washington Legal Foundation, a group funded by the Koch brothers.

After a courtroom scene in which the judges hammered both sides with questions and allowed them no time to answer, the justices voted 4 to 2 that the Board of Health had exceeded its authority. The four-judge majority had to go through logical contortions to get there, though. The board had inappropriately "legislated" because the rule required "choosing among competing policy goals," they wrote. At the same time, they agreed that the board *did* have the authority to "balance costs and benefits" when writing rules. And the board *had* acted within its authority when it passed rules banning lead paint in residences, requiring chain restaurants to post calorie labels, and requiring landlords to install window guards, because, they claimed, for these rules "the choices are not very difficult or complex."

The remaining two judges penned a scornful dissent. "There is no question that the Portion Cap Rule falls comfortably within the broad delegation granted to the board by the legislature," they wrote. "What petitioners have truly asked the courts to do is to strike down an *unpop-*

ular regulation, not an illegal one." The majority's decision to strike down the rule was little more than "camouflage for enforcement of judicial preferences."

It was our third loss over sugary drinks—the excise tax, the SNAP restriction, and now the portion cap—losses that bared the political and legal might of the soda companies. Staff in the health department were crushed. But we took solace that the department had begun something important. As Andy Goodman put it, "We put sugary drinks on the map" and pointed a finger at the soda companies as bearing some responsibility for obesity. "I think we fired a pretty big shot across their bow," said Tom Merrill. "We got the country and everybody talking about it." The many press stories on the battles effectively became counter-ads that gave sugary drinks an increasingly evil image.

In what mattered most, public health was winning. From 2007 to 2013, the fraction of adult New Yorkers saying that they drank sugary drinks daily fell by more than a third, from 36 to 23 percent, and the proportion of high school students drinking them dropped by more than a quarter, from 57 to 42 percent. Obesity rates in schoolchildren continued to edge down. And after rising from 2002 to 2012, the obesity rate in adult New Yorkers in 2013 dropped by a half percentage point. Maybe it was just a statistical fluke, or maybe it was a sign that the city had reached the high-water mark.

For all the health department's efforts, though, the food environment in New York City is still poisonous. Fast-food joints—many not part of any national chain—litter the city, pushing fried chicken and sodas. Grocery stores still load their highest-selling end aisles with bags of chips and huge bottles of sugar water. Even worse are the bodegas in poor neighborhoods. A typical one in Harlem sells bags of potato chips (120 calories and 2 grams of saturated fat) for 25 cents. A package of two Hostess cupcakes (360 calories) costs 50 cents. If you have only a quarter in your pocket, you can get a plain 4-ounce plastic bottle of sugar water. Or if you have two dollars, you can grab a 3-liter bottle of Tropical Fantasy Fruit Punch, flavored with "glycerol ester of wood rosin" and delivering 1,440 calories of high-fructose corn syrup. No wonder poor people suffer most from obesity and every other diet-related disease. Add to this junk food the power walls of cigarettes and the coolers of 40-ounce beer bottles, and bodegas look to me like toxic waste dumps. That is what comes to my mind when others ask if the Bloomberg administration overreached.

Obesity is now an epidemic around the world, with some countries rivaling the United States. From 1990 to 2010, as economies developed, the number of deaths globally from excess weight rose from fewer than those caused by childhood undernutrition to four times as many. In 2013 Kelly Henning at Bloomberg Philanthropies took the New York City obesity ideas to Mexico, where per capita sugary drink consumption was the world's highest. Compared to the trench warfare in New York, the Mexican campaign was a laser-guided-missile strike. Against fierce resistance by the soda companies, Mexican health advocates sprinted a bill through the legislature with taxes on soda and junk food. Early results of an evaluation of the soda tax by the Mexican National Institute of Public Health showed sugary drink purchases falling 10 percent, which is about what the studies that we used for New York's tax proposal predicted would happen.

The victory in Mexico washed back to the United States. In the November 2014 elections, voters in Berkeley, California, passed a referendum for a 1-cent-per-ounce soda tax by a three-to-one margin, despite the soda companies spending some $2.4 million—or $30 per voter—trying to block it. The Berkeley group won with a sophisticated political strategy that preempted the opponents' attacks, including signing on the NAACP as an early supporter and painting the soda companies as bad guys, even with their organization name: Berkeley vs. Big Soda. Bloomberg donated $650,000 to the tax campaign, and after the win, Howard Wolfson told reporters, "We stand ready to assess and assist other local efforts in the coming election cycle."

. . .

Mike Bloomberg began his years as mayor wanting to save lives millions at a time—but with no firm ideas about what public health would look like under him. Tom Frieden began his years as health commissioner with a goal to save as many New Yorkers' lives as possible, but with few firm ideas about how to attack tobacco or other major killers. That willingness to go wherever the data pointed them led both men into uncharted territory.

Often that territory was human behavior. The health department could save more lives by persuading New Yorkers to quit smoking, eat healthier food, and keep physically active than by giving them a cabinet full of medicines. Frieden and Bloomberg went there reluctantly. Frieden had come to the job believing in the life-saving potential of medicine, and Mary Bassett and Lynn Silver had to persuade him to join the fray in food policy. Bloomberg resisted meddling in personal choices but looked to his health commissioners to guide him and was unafraid to take a controversial action when he was convinced that it would save many lives.

The treacherous territory of human behavior was strikingly different from what New Yorkers expected the health department to occupy. When Tom Frieden spoke of obesity as an epidemic or said "trans fat kills," New Yorkers were puzzled and skeptical. Some viewed the health commissioner less as a savior than as an intrusion.

But human behavior is shaped by the world around us. Many of the behaviors that matter most to health involve consuming manufactured products—like cigarettes or soda—that are sold with aggressive corporate marketing. As Tom Frieden put it, defeating tobacco was much harder than defeating tuberculosis "because tuberculosis bacteria don't bribe politicians. They don't rebrand themselves as 'lite' bacteria. They don't hire movie stars to make it look cool to have tuberculosis." Battles with the corporations were inevitable. There was no way to reduce smoking in New York City without cutting into sales of cigarettes, prompting Philip Morris to fight back. There was no way to slow the obesity epidemic or fight heart disease without changing what New Yorkers ate and tangling with Burger King and Coca-Cola. People leading those corporations, even as they understood the dangers of their products, were obligated to resist because their shareholders demanded larger profits.

Most people view health work as genteel and generous, a gift from a kind-hearted person to those in need. But saving lives in America today means fighting to protect people from the pervasive marketing of cigarettes, junk food, and other unhealthy products. In New York City, those fights were worth it.

While the health department's clashes were always against companies, the press often framed them as battles against average people. New Yorkers didn't care about trans fats, but the press wrote that Mayor Bloomberg was taking away their French fries. Most New Yorkers endorsed smoke-free bars, but the press treated the Smoke-Free Air Act as a war on smokers. The press cast the battles as government versus citizen in part because the companies fed them that frame. A majority of New Yorkers initially supported "limiting the size of sugary drinks" sold in restaurants, but after the soda companies' public relations blitz, a majority opposed the attempt to "ban soda."

Battles like this required a different sort of health department. The health department of 1900 needed epidemiologists, microbiologists, sanitary engineers, inspectors, nurses, and doctors. The New York City health department of 2010 needed economists, lawyers, policy experts, data scientists, community activists, and specialists in using images and words in the mass media. During the Bloomberg years, Tom Frieden and I saw the New York City Department of Health and Mental Hygiene recreating itself for this new world.

Many who spoke to me for this book remembered their time at the health department as the highlight of their careers. Beth Kilgore, the media director for the antitobacco program, said, "I felt like we were the luckiest health department in the world because we got to really do things. . . . We've saved lives. We've done the right thing. We have done it for the right reasons. I mean, who can say that about their job?"

"It's such a powerhouse of a health department," said Tom Frieden. Winning public health victories with Mayor Bloomberg's support made its staff "fearless in terms of proposing and trying to get [more] things through." As Andy Goodman put it, "It was the coming together of the ideas and the political opportunity." The political opportunity needed ideas, but the ideas needed the political opportunity. Sarah Perl said, "Having done public health under Tom Frieden, at this particular moment in history, is a time that I will look back on in my old age and say 'You shoulda been there.'"

The reshaping of public health in New York City was contagious. During this period, the New York City Department of Health and Mental Hygiene became the organization that broke news and set a national agenda in public health. Staff from other health departments approached New Yorkers at national meetings to ask, "What's the next big thing?" New York's story will likely play out in similar ways elsewhere. I hope so, anyway.

Many of those who led the health department during the Bloomberg years have since taken their ideas to other leadership positions. After leaving New York, Tom Frieden became the nation's public health leader as director of the CDC. Farzad Mostashari was promoted to national coordinator for health information technology. Amanda Parsons and Susan Kansagra took charge of health promotion for big health care systems. Lynn Silver served as health officer for Sonoma County, California. In 2011 Sonia Angell took over as chief of noncommunicable diseases in the CDC's Center for Global Health. Mary Bassett, after working on health projects in Africa for the Doris Duke Charitable Foundation for four years, returned as New York City health commissioner under Bloomberg's successor, Bill de Blasio. When she returned, she brought back Coke McCord as an adviser and Sonia Angell as her deputy commissioner for chronic disease prevention. As of November 2014, most of the others I have featured in this book—including Tom Merrill, Sarah Perl, Beth Kilgore, Maura Kennelly, Christine Curtis, Kevin Schroth, Vicki Grimshaw, and Kelly Christ—continue to work for the New York City health department.

Good ideas in public health are not hard to find. The UN secretary-general is right that the greatest limit to our becoming much healthier is not a lack of ideas or even a lack of money. It is a shortage of leaders who are willing to take action to save lives in the face of determined opposition. As the British medical journal *Lancet* put it on its cover, "Of all

Michael Bloomberg's legacies to New York, lending his support to the gradual extension of human life may well prove the most meaningful of all." I hope that other elected officials will follow him.

Back at the United Nations, standing in front of the green marble desk, Mike Bloomberg summed up like this:

> First, we've learned that changing the social and physical environment is far more effective than changing individual behavior alone. . . .
>
> Second . . . healthy solutions are not necessarily costly solutions. Far from it. New York's Smoke-Free Air Act, our restrictions on trans fats, and our requirements concerning calorie posting in restaurants cost virtually nothing in public funds to implement. And raising cigarette taxes raises public revenues.
>
> Third, collaboration with the private sector . . . [is] very important. . . .
>
> But fourth and finally, while government action is not sufficient alone, it is nevertheless absolutely essential. There are powers only governments can exercise, policies only governments can mandate and enforce, and results only governments can achieve. To halt the worldwide epidemic of noncommunicable diseases, governments at all levels must make healthy solutions the default social option.
>
> That is, ultimately, government's highest duty.

Notes on Sources

The information in this book that didn't come from my memory came from interviews, health department documents (e-mails, notes from meetings, memoranda, reports, press releases), transcripts of public meetings, and press stories. I have listed the names of the persons I interviewed in my acknowledgments. Below are background and source documents that are publicly available but not easily found.

Chapter 1: *"Things are going to get really exciting."*

Tom Frieden spoke about his father and about "the single question that changed my life" in a TEDMED talk in 2012, at https://www.youtube.com/watch?v=rCBXijIXEdY.

Frieden's tuberculosis control work in New York City in the 1990s is summarized in T. R. Frieden et al., "Tuberculosis in New York City—Turning the Tide," *New England Journal of Medicine* 333 (1995): 229–33; and P. I. Fujiwara et al., "Directly Observed Therapy in New York City: History, Implementation, Results, and Challenges," *Clinics in Chest Medicine* 18 (1997): 135–48. His work in India is summarized in G. R. Khatri and T. R. Frieden, "Rapid DOTS Expansion in India," *Bulletin of the World Health Organization* 80 (2002): 457–63; and G. R. Khatri and T. R. Frieden, "Controlling Tuberculosis in India," *New England Journal of Medicine* 347 (2002): 1420–25.

Quotes from Michael Bloomberg during the 2001 mayoral campaign come from "Bloomberg Continues Retreat from Campaign Commercial," *New York Times,* June 17, 2001; "Bloomberg Raises His Profile and Promises a New Strategy," *New York Times,* September 27, 2001; "Being Mike Bloomberg, Without a

Script or a Doubt," *New York Times,* July 30, 2001; and "Bloomberg Says Education Can Prevent Illness," *New York Times,* July 19, 2001.

Health statistics for New York City are published in the health department's *Summary of Vital Statistics* series, at http://www.nyc.gov/html/doh/html/data/vs-summary.shtml.

The effects of cigarette taxes on smoking are reviewed in D. P. Hopkins et al., "Reviews of Evidence Regarding Interventions to Reduce Tobacco Use and Exposure to Environmental Tobacco Smoke," *American Journal of Preventive Medicine* 20, no. 2, supp. 1 (2001): 16–66. The price-sensitivity of teenagers is summarized in F. J. Chaloupka and Wechsler H. Price, "Tobacco Control Policies, and Smoking Among Young Adults," *Journal of Health Economics* 16 (1997): 359–73.

Articles on physician counseling to quit smoking include N. A. Rigotti, "Treatment of Tobacco Use and Dependence," *New England Journal of Medicine* 346 (2002): 506–12; and A. N. Thorndike, S. Regan, and N. A. Rigotti, "The Treatment of Smoking by US Physicians During Ambulatory Visits: 1994–2003," *American Journal of Public Health* 97 (2007): 1878–83. Figures on cessation counseling also come from Frieden's summaries of the research and his estimates in 2002.

The risks of secondhand smoke are summarized in the U.S. Surgeon General's report *The Health Consequences of Involuntary Exposure to Tobacco Smoke* (Atlanta: Centers for Disease Control and Prevention, 2006), available at http://www.surgeongeneral.gov/library/reports. Research on the effect of indoor smoking bans is summarized in appendix B-2 of Hopkins et al., "Reviews of Evidence Regarding Interventions to Reduce Tobacco Use." The effect of home smoking bans is described in J. P. Pierce et al., *Tobacco Control in California: Who's Winning the War? An Evaluation of the Tobacco Control Program, 1989–1996* (La Jolla: University of California at San Diego, 1998) and is summarized in R. C. Brownson et al., "Effects of Smoking Restrictions in the Workplace," *Annual Review of Public Health* 23 (2002): 333–48.

Chapter 2: *"I need a one-pager on lives saved."*

On the history of the New York City health department, see John Duffy, *A History of Public Health in New York City, 1625–1866* (New York: Russell Sage Foundation, 1968), and *A History of Public Health in New York City, 1866–1966* (New York: Russell Sage Foundation, 1974). A short summary is *Protecting Public Health in New York City: 200 Years of Leadership* (New York City Department of Health and Mental Hygiene, 2005), available at http://www.nyc.gov/health.

Coke McCord's article on mortality in Harlem is C. McCord and H. P.

Freeman, "Excess Mortality in Harlem," *New England Journal of Medicine* 322 (1990): 173–77.

The risks of secondhand smoke in restaurants and bars are discussed in M. Siegel, "Involuntary Smoking in the Restaurant Workplace: A Review of Employee Exposure and Health Effects," *Journal of the American Medical Association* 270 (1993): 490–93; and J. P. Leigh, "Occupations, Cigarette Smoking, and Lung Cancer in the Epidemiological Follow-Up to the NHANES I and the California Occupational Mortality Study," *Bulletin of the New York Academy of Medicine* 73 (1996): 370–97.

Data on employment and sales in bars and restaurants in California in the late 1990s were obtained from the state's Employment Development Department and the California Board of Equalization, respectively.

Chapter 3: *"I thought, this nutrition stuff is so controversial."*

Mary Bassett's short autobiography is in M. T. Bassett, "From Harlem to Harare," in Anne-Emanuelle Birn and Theodore M. Brown, eds., *Comrades in Health: U.S. Health Internationalists, Abroad and at Home* (New Brunswick, NJ: Rutgers University Press, 2013).

Geoffrey Rose's curves appear in his book *The Strategy of Preventive Medicine* (Oxford: Oxford University Press, 1994).

The chemistry and history of trans fats are described in W. Shurtleff and A. Aoyagi, "History of Soy Oil Hydrogenation and of Research on the Safety of Hydrogenated Vegetable Oils," available at http://www.thesoydailyclub.com/SFC/MSPproducts501.asp. The health effects of trans fats are described in *Letter Report on Dietary Reference Intakes of Trans Fatty Acids* (National Academy of Sciences, Institute of Medicine, 2002), available at http://mem.iom.edu/CMS/5410/13083 .aspx. Other articles include D. Mozaffarian et al., "Trans Fatty Acids and Cardiovascular Disease," *New England Journal of Medicine* 354 (2006): 1601–13; D. B. Allison et al., "Estimated Intakes of Trans Fatty and Other Fatty Acids in the US Population," *Journal of the American Dietetic Association* 99 (1999): 166–74; and W. C. Willett and A. Ascherio, "Trans Fatty Acids: Are the Effects Only Marginal?" *American Journal of Public Health* 84 (1994): 722–24.

The health department's nicotine patch distribution program is summarized in N. Miller et al., "Effectiveness of a Large-Scale Distribution Programme of Free Nicotine Patches: A Prospective Evaluation," *Lancet* 365 (2005):1849–54.

The telephone survey started by Farzad Mostashari was called the Community Health Survey, and its annual results can be queried through the health department's EpiQuery tool at https://a816-healthpsi.nyc.gov/epiquery.

Information about the first-year impact of the Smoke-Free Air Act appears in the health department's *The State of Smoke-Free New York City: A One-Year Review*, available at http://www.nyc.gov/html/doh/downloads/pdf/smoke/sfaa-2004report .pdf. Revenue from the city's cigarette tax can be found in the Comprehensive Annual Financial Report of the Comptroller, available at http://comptroller.nyc .gov/reports/comprehensive-annual-financial-reports. The academic article on the Smoke-Free Air Act is C. Chang et al., "The New York City Smoke-Free Air Act: Second-Hand Smoke as a Worker Health and Safety Issue," *American Journal of Industrial Medicine* 46 (2004): 188–95, and the article summarizing the early success of smoking program is T. R. Frieden et al., "Adult Tobacco Use Measures After Intensive Tobacco Control Measures," *American Journal of Public Health* 95 (2005): 1016–23.

The entire New York City Health Code is available at http://www.nyc.gov/ html/doh/html/about/health-code.shtml, and the City Charter at http://www .nyc.gov/html/charter/downloads/pdf/citycharter2004.pdf.

Chapter 4: *"We were failing and we didn't know why, and we had to succeed."*

The effect of the FTC's application of the Fairness Doctrine to cigarette advertising is described in K. E. Warner, "The Effects of the Antismoking Campaign on Cigarette Consumption," *American Journal of Public Health* 67 (1977): 645–50, and in chapter 12 of National Cancer Institute, *The Role of the Media in Promoting and Reducing Tobacco Use*, Tobacco Control Monograph no. 19 (Washington, DC: U.S. Department of Health and Human Services, National Institutes of Health, 2008), which also summarizes the evaluations of antismoking campaigns described in the chapter. Many of the antismoking ads that the health department ran beginning in 2006 are on the World Lung Foundation's website http://www .worldlungfoundation.org. The department's early ad campaign and the smoking trends after them are summarized in J. A. Ellis et al., "Decline in Smoking Prevalence—New York City, 2002–2006," *Morbidity and Mortality Weekly Report* 56 (2007): 604–8.

Results of Quinnipiac University's polls of mayoral approval are at http:// www.quinnipiac.edu/news-and-events/quinnipiac-university-poll/new-york-city.

The Americans for Nonsmokers' Rights posts data and reports on smoke-free laws at www.no-smoke.org. An early story on smoking bans in Europe is "Antitobacco Trend Has Reached Europe," *New York Times*, August 11, 2003.

Much of Tom Frieden's original proposal for global tobacco control is contained in the slide set *How to Prevent 100 Million Deaths from Tobacco*, at www.globaltobaccocontrol.org/node/11045, and in T. R. Frieden and M. R. Bloomberg, "How to Prevent 100 Million Deaths from Tobacco," *Lancet* 369 (2007): 1758–61. The announcement is summarized in a press release at http://www.tobaccofreekids.org/pressoffice/BloombergRelease.pdf and in "Where There's Smoke There's Ire, and the Mayor's Cash," *New York Times*, August 16, 2006.

Chapter 5: *"Are you sure this will save lives?"*

Early press reports on trans fats include "Hold That Fat, New York Asks Its Restaurants," *New York Times*, August 11, 2005; "The Panic Du Jour: Trans Fats in Foods," *New York Times*, August 14, 2005; and "Grease and Desist: City Eateries Told to Upgrade Oils," *New York Post*, August 11, 2005.

On the growth of the obesity epidemic, see K. M. Flegal et al., "Prevalence and Trends in Obesity Among U.S. Adults, 1999–2000," *Journal of the American Medical Association* 288 (2002): 1723–27; and C. L. Ogden et al., "Prevalence of Overweight and Obesity in the United States, 1999–2004," *Journal of the American Medical Association* 296 (2006): 1549–55. On deaths associated with obesity, see K. M. Flegal et al., "Excess Deaths Associated with Underweight, Overweight, and Obesity," *Journal of the American Medical Association* 293 (2005): 1861–67. Trends in portion sizes from the 1970s to the 1990s are described in S. J. Nielsen and B. M. Popkin, "Patterns and Trends in Food Portion Sizes, 1977–1998," *Journal of the American Medical Association* 289 (2003): 450–53.

On Americans' perceptions of their weight and attempts to lose weight, see V. W. Chang and N. A. Christakis, "Self-perception of Weight Appropriateness in the United States," *American Journal of Preventive Medicine* 24 (2003): 332–39; and J. Kruger et al., "Attempting to Lose Weight: Specific Practices Among U.S. Adults," *American Journal of Preventive Medicine* 26 (2004): 402–6. On how accurately people estimate calories, see S. Burton et al., "Attacking the Obesity Epidemic: The Potential Health Benefits of Providing Nutrition Information at Restaurants," *American Journal of Public Health* 96 (2006): 1669–75; and J. R. Backstrand et al., "Fat Chance: a Survey of Dietitians' Knowledge of Calories and Fat in Restaurant Meals," available at portionteller.com/pdf/cspistudy97.pdf.

For more on the health department's trans fat work, see S. Y. Angell et al., "Cholesterol Control Beyond the Clinic: New York City's Trans Fat Restriction," *Annals of Internal Medicine* 151 (2009): 129–34.

Initial reactions to the trans fat proposal are described in "New York City Plans Limits on Restaurants' Use of Trans Fats," *New York Times*, September 27, 2006; "Some Owners Uneasy About Proposal," *New York Times*, September 27, 2006; "Don't Let Them Eat Cake," *New York Post*, September 28, 2006; and "Goodbye Fries? NYC May Ban Trans Fats," Associated Press, September 26, 2006. The quotes from Applebee's and from the National Restaurant Association (about the effect of a trans fat ban on traffic and congestion) come from their written comments to the Board of Health, which were summarized in a memorandum from the health department staff to Tom Frieden for the attention of the board, available at http://www.nyc.gov/html/doh/downloads/pdf/cardio/cardio-transfat-comments-response.pdf. Dunkin' Brands efforts to eliminate trans fats are described in "The Long, Secret Journey to a Healthier Donut," *Boston Globe*, September 16, 2007. An article about the food industry's opposition is "McDonald's Readies for NYC Trans Fat Fight," *Crain's New York Business*, November 14, 2006.

Chapter 6: *"I just went on a field trip to Dunkin' Donuts."*

More detail on the calorie-labeling rule appears in T. A. Farley et al., "New York City's Fight Over Calorie Labeling," *Health Affairs* 28 (2009): 1098–109. The final rule appears in section 81.50 of the Health Code, http://www.nyc.gov/html/doh/html/about/health-code.shtml.

The study on the relationship between supermarket availability and obesity is K. Moreland et al., "Supermarkets, Other Food Stores, and Obesity," *American Journal of Preventive Medicine* 30 (2006): 333–39.

The transcript of the committee on consumer affairs' hearing on Green Carts on January 31, 2008, is posted on the City Council's website at http://legistar.council.nyc.gov/Calendar.aspx. The initiative is the subject of the documentary *The Apple Pushers*, http://www.applepushers.com.

The Marie series of antismoking ads are posted on the DCF website http://www.dcfadvertising.com.

Chapter 7: *"Now, for the first time ever, she could see for herself."*

The article on the low quality of medical care in the United States is E. A. McGlynn et al., "The Quality of Health Care Delivered to Adults in the United States," *New England Journal of Medicine* 348 (2003): 2635–45.

The health department's public health detailing work is summarized in K. Larson et al., "Public Health Detailing: A Strategy to Improve the Delivery of Clinical Preventive Services in New York City," *Public Health Reports* 12 (2006): 228–34.

The clinical decision support system for the Primary Care Information Project is described in S. Amirfar et al., "Developing Public Health Clinical Decision Support Systems (CDSS) for the Outpatient Community in New York City: Our Experience," *BMC Public Health* 11 (2011): 753.

Farzad Mostashari described the health department's program to get doctors using its electronic medical records in F. Mostashari, M. Tripathi, and M. Kendall, "A Tale of Two Large Community Electronic Health Record Extension Projects," *Health Affairs* 28 (2009): 354–56.

The Australian antismoking ad *Separation* is posted on the World Lung Foundation's website http://www.worldlungfoundation.org.

Chapter 8: *"There's no doubt our kids drink way too much soda."*

The history of dietary guidelines on fat is summarized in K. D. Gifford, "Dietary Fats, Eating Guides, and Public Policy: History, Critique, and Recommendations," *American Journal of Medicine* 113, no. 9, supp. 2 (2002): 89–106. The trends toward increasing carbohydrate intake are included in R. R. Briefel and C. L. Johnson, "Secular Trends in Dietary Intake in the United States," *Annual Review of Nutrition* 24 (2004): 401–31. An article rethinking the focus on fat is D. S. Ludwig, "Dietary Glycemic Index and Obesity," *Journal of Nutrition* 130, no. 2 (2000): 280S–283S. Gary Taubes's article on the risks of fats and carbohydrates is "What If It's All Been a Big Fat Lie?," *New York Times Magazine*, July 7, 2002. The study on teenagers that supports the hypothesis about the glycemic index is D. S. Ludwig et al., "High Glycemic Index Foods Overeating, and Obesity," *Pediatrics* 103 (1999): e26.

Robert Lustig's articles on the toxicity of sugar include R. H. Lustig, "The Toxic Truth About Sugar," *Nature,* February 2, 2012, and R. H. Lustig, "Fructose: Metabolic, Hedonic, and Societal Parallels with Ethanol," *Journal of the American Dietetic Association* 110 (2010): 1307–21.

Studies on the satiety of liquid versus solid food are R. Mattes, "Fluid Calories and Energy Balance: The Good, the Bad, and the Uncertain," *Physiology and Behavior* 89 (2006): 66–70; and D. P. DiMeglio and R. D. Mattes, "Liquid Versus Solid Carbohydrate: Effects on Food Intake and Body Weight," *International Journal of Obesity* 24 (2000): 794–800.

Studies on sugary drinks and obesity include M. B. Schulze et al., "Sugar-sweetened Beverages, Weight Gain, and Incidence of Type 2 Diabetes in Young and Middle-Aged Women," *Journal of the American Medical Association* 292 (2004): 927–34; and V. S. Malik, M. B. Schulze, and F. B. Hu, "Intake of Sugar-Sweetened Beverages and Weight Gain: A Systematic Review," *American Journal of Clinical Nutrition* 84 (2006): 274–88. Studies tracking the rise in sugary drink consumption include S. J. Nielsen et al., "Trends in Energy Intake in United States Between 1977 and 1996: Similar Shifts Seen Across Age Groups," *Obesity Research* 10 (2002): 370–78; S. J. Nielsen et al., "Changes in Beverage Intake Between 1977 and 2001," *American Journal of Preventive Medicine* 27 (2004): 205–10; B. K. Kit et al., "Trends in Sugar-Sweetened Beverage Consumption Among Youth and Adults in the United States: 1999–2010," *American Journal of Clinical Nutrition* 98 (2013): 180–88; and R. K. Johnson et al., "Dietary Sugars Intake and Cardiovascular Health," *Circulation* 120 (2009): 1011–20.

The potential effect of a tax on sugary drinks, as measured by the price elasticity, is discussed in T. Andreyeva et al., "The Impact of Food Prices on Consumption: A Systematic Review of Research on the Price Elasticity of Demand for Food," *American Journal of Public Health* 100 (2010): 216–22.

An article mentioning Indra Nooyi's trouble with investors over straying from the unhealthiest items is "Pepsi Chief Shuffles Management to Soothe Investors," *New York Times* March 12, 2012.

To evaluate the effect of calorie labeling on menus, the health department conducted surveys of purchases at fast-food restaurants in New York City. The first surveys were completed in 2007, before the calorie labels appeared. Analyses appear in M. T. Bassett et al., "Purchasing Behavior and Calorie Information at Fast-Food Chains in New York City, 2007," *American Journal of Public Health* 98 (2008): 1457–59; T. Dumanovsky et al., "What People Buy from Fast-Food Restaurants: Caloric Content and Menu Item Selection, New York City, 2007," *Obesity* 17 (2009): 1369–74; and C. Huang et al., "Calories from Beverages Purchased at 2 Major Coffee Chains in New York City, 2007," *Preventing Chronic Disease* 6 (2009): A118.

Some articles that appeared after the calorie labels went up are "Restaurants That Lack Calorie Counts Now Face Fines," *New York Times,* July 19, 2008; "Running from Dunkin'," *New York Sun,* June 24, 2008; "NYC Chain Restaurants Posting Calories on Menus," Reuters.com, July 20, 2008; and "On the Table: The Calories Lurking in Restaurant Food," *Wall Street Journal,* July 29, 2008. Dunkin' Donuts' lower-calorie sandwiches are described in "Dunkin' Donuts to Offer Healthier Menu Items," Associated Press, July 30, 2008.

The poll on obesity policy was conducted by Lake, Snell, Perry & Associates in 2003 and the report is available at http://www.phsi.harvard.edu/health_reform/poll_results.pdf.

The changes to school food in New York City during the Bloomberg years are summarized in S. E. Perlman et al., "A Menu for Health: Changes to New York City School Food, 2001–2011," *Journal of School Health* 82 (2012): 484–91.

Obesity in children in Head Start programs is discussed in C. L. Williams et al., "Body Size and Cardiovascular Risk Factors in a Preschool Population," *Preventive Cardiology* 7 (2004): 116–21.

City government nutrition standards and the process of developing them are described in A. Lederer et al., "Toward a Healthier City: Nutrition Standards for New York City Government," *American Journal of Preventive Medicine* 46 (2014): 423–28. The standards themselves are available at http://www.nyc.gov/html/doh/html/living/agency-food-standards.shtml.

School snack vending policies around the country in the early 2000s are summarized in the Center for Science in the Public Interest's "School Foods Report Card 2007," available at http://www.cspinet.org/2007schoolreport.pdf. The announcement of Clinton's soda agreement is summarized in "Soda Distributors to End Most School Sales," *Washington Post*, May 3, 2006.

Initial reactions to Paterson's soda tax proposal are described in "A Tax on Many Soft Drinks Sets Off a Spirited Debate," *New York Times*, December 17, 2008, and the discussion continued in articles such as K. D. Brownell and T. R. Frieden, "Ounces of Prevention—The Public Policy Case for Taxes on Sugared Beverages," *New England Journal of Medicine* 360 (2009): 1805–8; "Sodas a Tempting Target," *New York Times*, May 20, 2009; "Tax Proposals Draw Critics in Talks on Financing Health Insurance," *New York Times*, May 21, 2009; K. D. Brownell et al., "The Public Health and Economic Benefits of Taxing Sugar-Sweetened Beverages," *New England Journal of Medicine* 361 (2009): 1599–605; and "Dr. Tom's Toughest Case," *New York Post,* September 12, 2009. Stephen Colbert's rant on the topic on May 12, 2009, is at http://thecolbertreport.cc.com/videos/vyychn/stephen-s-coke-party-protest.

Chapter 9: *"In the end, it's just ketchup."*

An article that ranks hypertension relative to other major health risks is G. Danaei et al., "The Preventable Causes of Death in the United States: Comparative Risk Assessment of Dietary, Lifestyle, and Metabolic Risk Factors," *PLoS Medicine* 6 (2009): e100058.

Salt: The Forgotten Killer is available at http://www.cspinet.org/salt. A review of the risks of salt is F. J. He and G. A. MacGregor, "A Comprehensive Review on Salt and Health and Current Experience of Worldwide Salt Reduction Programs," *Journal of Human Hypertension* 23 (2009): 363–84. The benefit of low-salt diets was shown in F. M. Sacks et al., "Effect on Blood Pressure of Reduced Sodium and the Dietary Approaches to Stop Hypertension (DASH) Diet," *New England Journal of Medicine* 344 (2001): 3–10.

Some key articles on the INTERSALT study are "INTERSALT: An International Study of Electrolyte Excretion and Blood Pressure. Results for 24-Hour Urinary Sodium and Potassium Excretion," *British Medical Journal* 297 (1988): 319–30, and J. J. M. Carvalho et al., "Blood Pressure in Four Remote Populations in the INTERSALT Study," *Hypertension* 14 (1989): 238–46.

Estimates of salt consumption during the Paleolithic period appear in M. Konner and S. B. Eaton, "Paleolithic Nutrition: Twenty-Five Years Later," *Nutrition in Clinical Practice* 25 (2010): 594–602.

The health benefits of reducing sodium intake are estimated in K. Palar and R. Sturm, "Potential Societal Savings from Reduced Sodium Consumption in the U.S. Adult Population," *American Journal of Health Promotion* 24 (2009): 49–57.

Information on the sources of sodium in the American diet can be found in R. D. Mattes, "Relative Contributions of Dietary Sodium Sources," *Journal of the American College of Nutrition* 10 (1991): 383–93; and in a Web appendix to P. A. Cotton et al., "Dietary Sources of Nutrients Among U.S. Adults, 1994–1996, "*Journal of the American Dietetic Association* 104 (2004): 921–30.

The change in salt preference from eating less salt is described in M. Bertino et al., "Long-term Reductions in Dietary Sodium Alters the Taste of Salt," *American Journal of Clinical Nutrition* 36 (1982): 1134–44.

The Finland success story on salt is described in H. Karppanen and E. Mervaala, "Sodium Intake and Hypertension," *Progress in Cardiovascular Disease* 49 (2006): 59–75; and T. Laatikainen et al., "Sodium in the Finnish Diet: 20-Year Trends in Urinary Sodium Among the Adult Population," *European Journal of Clinical Nutrition* 60 (2006): 965–70.

Failed efforts on sodium in the United States appear in a report on the 1969 White House Conference on Food, Nutrition and Health, available at http://www.nns.nih.gov/1969/full_report/White_House_Report2_S2.pdf; and A. H. Hayes, Jr., "FDA's Dietary Sodium Initiative—In the War Against Hypertension, a New Weapon," *Public Health Reports* 98 (1983): 207–10. Trends in sodium intake in the United States are available in R. R. Briefel and C. L. Johnson, "Secular Trends in Dietary Intake in the United States," *Annual Review of Nutrition* 24 (2004): 401–31.

The work of the United Kingdom's Food Standards Agency to reduce salt in foods is described in a report available at http://www.food.gov.uk/sites/default/files/multimedia/pdfs/saltreductioninitiatives.pdf.

The study on saltshakers is G. K. Beauchamp et al., "Failure to Compensate Decreased Dietary Sodium with Increased Table Salt Usage," *Journal of the American Medical Association* 258 (1987): 3275–78.

Early reports on the nH1N1 epidemic are "Fighting Deadly Flu Outbreak, Mexico Shuts Schools or Millions," *New York Times,* April 25, 2009; and "Health Officials Investigate Illness at Queens Private School," *New York Times*, April 25, 2009.

Chapter 10: *"All I could think of was, welcome to New York."*

Americans for Nonsmokers' Rights maintains data and compiles reports on smoke-free laws, which are available at http://www.no-smoke.org. For more on the spread of smoke-free air rules in Europe, see "Europe's 'No Smoking' Zones," *Independent,* January 5, 2006; and "French Smoking Ban: The End of a Way of Life?," *New York Times,* January 1, 2008.

Chapter 11: *"They can't even be bothered to sue us?"*

The Federal Trade Commission issues annual reports on how tobacco companies spend their billions promoting smoking. They are available at http://www.ftc.gov/industry/tobacco.

Americans for Nonsmokers' Rights maintains a list of municipalities with smoke-free parks at http://www.no-smoke.org. A study on the smoke generated by cigarettes outdoors is N. E. Klepeis et al., "Real-time Measurement of Outdoor Tobacco Smoke Particles," *Journal of the Air and Waste Management Association* 57 (2007): 522–34. Other researchers showed that people exposed to tobacco smoke outdoors had elevated levels of cotinine: see J. C. Hall et al., "Assessment of Exposure to Secondhand Smoke at Outdoor Bars and Family Restaurants in Athens, Georgia, Using Salivary Cotinine," *Journal of Occupational and Environmental Hygiene* 6 (2009): 698–704.

Chapter 12: *"We were outgunned."*

Studies on the effect of menu calorie labeling are B. Elbel et al., "Calorie Labeling and Food Choices: A First Look at the Effect on Low-Income People in New York City," *Health Affairs* 2009: w1110–21; T. Dumanovsky et al., "Consumer Awareness of Fast-Food Calorie Information in New York City After Implementation of a Menu Labeling Regulation," *American Journal of Public Health* 100 (2010): 2520–25; T. Dumanovsky et al., "Changes in Energy Content of Lunchtime Purchases from Fast Food Restaurants After Introduction of Calorie Labeling: Cross-Sectional Customer Surveys," *British Medical Journal* 343 (2011): d4464; and G. Bollinger et al., "Calorie Posting in Chain Restaurants," NBER Working Paper No. 15648, available at http://www.nber.org.

The health department's *Pouring on the Pounds* ads (including *Man Drinking Fat*) are posted at http://www.nyc.gov/html/doh/html/living/sugarydrink-media-archive.shtml.

An ad promoting the soda tax in 2010 is posted at https://www.youtube.com/watch?v=ucABebGFms0. Ads against it are at https://www.youtube.com/watch?v=qXg0RTquFwc and https://www.youtube.com/watch?v=UtuvB20HXbs.

Data on federal lobbying contributions by Coca-Cola, PepsiCo, and the American Beverage Association are available from the Office of the Clerk, U.S. House of Representatives, at http://lobbyingdisclosure.house.gov. Articles on their contributions to state legislators include "Lobbyists Targeted Westchester Pols to Make Soda Tax Idea Go Flat," *Daily News*, March 26, 2010; "Soda Tax Seems to Be Falling Flat," *Albany Times-Union,* March 16, 2010; and "Drink Makers Lead $211M Lobby Gusher," *New York Post*, March 5, 2011. A postmortem of the tax attempt is "Failure of State Soda Tax Plan Reflects Power of an Antitax Message," *New York Times*, July 3, 2010.

Chapter 13: *"Would you like us to say, 'That's not our responsibility'?"*

Initial press reports on the National Salt Reduction Initiative include "One Family's Diet Full of Hidden Salt," *Daily News*, January 12, 2010; "New York Seeks National Effort to Curtail Salt Use," *New York Times*, January 11, 2010; and "Food Makers Quietly Cut Back on Salt," *Wall Street Journal*, January 11, 2010. Jane Brody's column is "After Smoking and Fats, Focus Turns to Salt," *New York Times*, January 26, 2010. The Quinnipiac poll on New York City's food initiatives is available at http://www.quinnipiac.edu/news-and-events/quinnipiac-university-poll/new-york-city/release-detail?ReleaseID=1425.

Michael Alderman's commentary on salt is "Reducing Dietary Sodium: The Case for Caution," *Journal of the American Medical Association* 303 (2010): 448–49. His affiliation with the Salt Institute is mentioned briefly at the end of this article.

The final National Salt Reduction Targets and the company commitments to meet them are available at http://www.nyc.gov/html/doh/html/diseases/salt.shtml. For the companies' announcements of their salt reduction commitments, see "Salt Taking a Cut in Groceries, Restaurant Menus," Associated Press, April 26, 2010; and "Salt Assault Gets Allies," *Wall Street Journal*, April 26, 2010.

The report from the Institute of Medicine is J. E. Henney, C. L. Taylor, and

C. S. Boon, eds., *Strategies to Reduce Sodium Intake in the United States* (Washington, DC: National Academies Press, 2010).

The study showing the improvement in quality of care with the electronic medical records is S. C. Shih et al., "Health Information Systems in Small Practices: Improving the Delivery of Clinical Preventive Services," *American Journal of Preventive Medicine* 41 (2011): 603–9.

Chapter 14: *"We are in a coalition with major food companies for one reason only; that is, access to power."*

Background on SNAP is available at http://www.snaptohealth.org, and data on the program is at http://www.fns.usda.gov/sites/default/files/pd/SNAPsummary .pdf. The history of the program is described in P. S. Landers, "The Food Stamp Program: History, Nutrition, Education, and Impact," *Journal of the American Dietetic Association* 107 (2007): 1945–51.

The effects of the WIC changes on the foods that stores stocked and children's diets are presented in T. Andreyeva et al., "Positive Influence of the Revised Special Supplemental Nutrition Program for Women, Infants, and Children Food Packages on Access to Healthy Foods," *Journal of the Academy of Nutrition and Dietetics* 112 (2012): 850–58; A. Hillier et al., "The Impact of WIC Food Package Changes on Access to Healthful Food in 2 Low-Income Urban Neighborhoods," *Journal of Nutrition Education and Behavior* 44, no. 3 (2012): 210–16; A. Kong et al., "The 18-month Impact of Special Supplemental Nutrition Program for Women Infants and Children Food Package Revisions on Diets of Recipient Families," *American Journal of Preventive Medicine* 46 (2014): 543–51; and S. E. Whaley et al., "Revised WIC Food Package Improves Diet in WIC Families," *Journal of Nutrition Education and Behavior* 44 (2012): 204–9.

Edward Cooney's comment on the Congressional Hunger Center's ties to the major food companies is in "Let Them Eat Broccoli," *New York Times*, October 17, 2010.

On the health department e-mails on the ten-pound claim, see "E-mails Reveal Dispute Over the City's Ad Against Sodas," *New York Times*, October 29, 2010. The editorial mentioned is "Farley's Big Fat Lie," *New York Post*, October 30, 2010.

On the body converting glucose into fat, see L. H. Glimcher and A.-H. Lee, "From Sugar to Fat," *Annals of the New York Academy of Sciences* 1173, supp. 1 (2009): E2–E9. The study of the effect of overfeeding on weight gain is C. Bouchard et al., "The Response to Long-Term Overfeeding in Identical Twins," *New England Journal of Medicine* 322 (1990): 1477–82.

Barbara Rolls's study on the portion size of macaroni and cheese is B. J. Rolls et al., "Portion Size of Food Affects Energy Intake in Normal-Weight and Overweight Men and Women," *American Journal of Clinical Nutrition* 76 (2002): 1207–13. Other studies on the effects of portion size include B. J. Rolls et al., "Increasing the Portion Size of a Sandwich Increases Energy Intake," *Journal of the American Dietetic Association* 104 (2004): 367–72; B. J. Rolls et al., "Increasing the Portion Size of a Packaged Snack Increases Energy Intake in Men and Women," *Appetite* 42 (2004): 63–69; K. C. Mathias et al., "Serving Larger Portions of Fruits and Vegetables Together at Dinner Promotes Intake of Both Foods in Young Children," *Journal of the Academy of Nutrition and Dietetics* 112 (2012): 266–70; J. E. Flood et al., "The Effect of Increased Beverage Portion Size on Energy Intake at a Meal," *Journal of the American Dietetic Association* 106 (2006): 1984–90; and B. J. Rolls et al., "The Effect of Large Portion Sizes on Energy Intake Is Sustained for 11 Days," *Obesity* 15 (2007): 1535–43.

Brian Wansink's self-refilling bowl study is B. Wansink et al., "Bottomless Bowls: Why Visual Cues of Portion Size May Influence Intake," *Obesity Research* 13 (2005): 93–100.

A study on the growth of portion sizes in fast-food restaurants is L. R. Young and M. Nestle, "Expanding Portion Size in the US Marketplace: Implications for Nutrition Counseling," *Journal of the American Dietetic Association* 103 (2003): 231–34. More information is in L. Young, *The Portion Teller Plan: The No-Diet Reality Guide to Eating, Cheating, and Losing Weight Permanently* (New York: Morgan Road Books, 2005). A study on the growth of portion sizes overall is S. J. Nielsen and B. M. Popkin, "Patterns and Trends in Food Portion Sizes," *Journal of the American Medical Association* 289 (2003): 450–53.

Chapter 15: *"They always had two nuclear weapons."*

The *Suffering Every Minute of Every Day* ads are posted on the World Lung Foundation's website http://www.worldlungfoundation.org.

Data on life expectancy in New York City during this period are included in the health department's annual *Summary of Vital Statistics* and in a March 2013 *Epi Research Report* entitled "Increased Life Expectancy in New York City: What Accounts for the Gains?," both of which are available at http://www.nyc.gov/health.

Information on marketing expenditures by the tobacco companies, including those for point-of-purchase displays, is in the annual *Federal Trade Commission Cigarette Report* available at http://www.ftc.gov. The surveys of smokers leaving retail outlets are summarized in O. B. Carter et al., "The Effect of Retail Cigarette Pack Displays on Unplanned Purchases: Results from Immediate Postpurchase Interviews," *Tobacco Control* 18 (2009): 218–21. Studies of the effect of point-of-purchase displays on children include M. Wakefield et al., "An Experimental Study of Effects on Schoolchildren of Exposure to Point-of-Sale Cigarette Advertising and Pack Displays," *Health Education Research* 21 (2006): 338–47; T. Dewhirst, "POP Goes the Power Wall? Taking Aim at Tobacco Promotional Strategies Utilized at Retail," *Tobacco Control* 13 (2004): 209–10; and L. Henriksen et al., "Effects on Youth of Exposure to Retail Tobacco Advertising," *Journal of Applied Social Psychology* 32 (2002): 1771–89. The prospective study from Stanford is L. Henriksen et al., "A Longitudinal Study of Exposure to Retail Cigarette Advertising and Smoking Initiation," *Pediatrics* 126 (2010): 232–38.

The *Framework Convention on Tobacco Control* is accessible at the World Health Organization's website http://www.who.int/fctc.

Youth smoking rates in Ontario after the tobacco product display ban was put into effect (from 2008 to 2009) are available from the annual Youth Smoking Survey results on the Health Canada website at http://www.hc-sc.gc.ca.

The Supreme Court case on the Vermont law on prescribing patterns of physicians is *Sorrell v. IMS Health Inc.*, no. 10-779 131 S.Ct. 2653 (2011).

The opinion about the legality of a product display ban is discussed in M. Berman, M. Miura, and J. Bergstresser, *Tobacco Product Display Restrictions* (Boston: Center for Public Health and Tobacco Policy at New England Law, 2010), available at http://publichealthlawcenter.org.

The virtual reality study on tobacco product displays is A. E. Kim et al., "Influence of Tobacco Displays and Ads on Youth: A Virtual Store Experiment," *Pediatrics* 131 (2013): 1–8.

The expenditures for price discounts for cigarettes is contained table 2D of the Federal Trade Commission's *Cigarette Report* for 2011, available at http://www.ftc.gov.

Chapter 16: *"I hear that your mayor wants to ban soda!"*

The health department's EpiQuery data analysis tool, available at http://nyc.gov/health or https://a816-healthpsi.nyc.gov/epiquery, can be used to view results from the department's annual telephone surveys, which include questions on obesity and sugary drink consumption.

A report on the declines in childhood obesity in New York City was published in the CDC newsletter: M. Berger et al., "Obesity in K-8 students—

New York City, 2006–07 to 2010–11 school years," *Morbidity and Mortality Weekly Report* 60 (2011): 1673–78.

The first stories on the portion cap were "Mayor Bloomberg Wants to Impose 16-Ounce Limit on Sugar Drinks," *New York Post*, May 31, 2012; and "New York Plans to Ban Sale of Big Sizes of Sugary Drinks," *New York Times*, May 30, 2012. The poll about this proposal was done by Quinnipiac University, and the results were posted on its website on June 13, 2012.

The Million Big Gulp March rally was described in "A Rally for Sweet-Drink Rights Comes Soaked in Patriotism," *New York Times,* July 23, 2012. A promotional video made by the public relations firm is posted at https://www.youtube.com/watch?v=ctAiZ0w8YCI.

Chapter 17: *"The NSRI's success is far from guaranteed."*

The Center for Science in the Public Interest's report on changes in salt in foods is M. F. Jacobson et al., "Changes in Sodium Levels in Processed and Restaurant Foods, 2005 to 2011," *JAMA Internal Medicine* 173 (2013): 1285–91. The editorial on the National Salt Reduction Initiative is S. Y. Angell and T. A. Farley, "Can We Finally Make Progress on Sodium Intake?" *American Journal of Public Health* 102 (2012): 1625–27.

The articles on sodium and mortality mentioned in the chapter are K. Stolarz-Skrzpek et al., "Fatal and Nonfatal Outcomes, Incidence of Hypertension, and Blood Pressure Changes in Relation to Urinary Sodium Excretion," *Journal of the American Medical Association* 305 (2011): 1777–85; and M. J. O'Donnell et al., "Urinary Sodium and Potassium Excretion and Risk of Cardiovascular Events," *Journal of the American Medical Association* 306 (2011): 2229–38. Examples of comments criticizing these studies are D. R. Labarthe and P. A. Briss, "Urinary Sodium Excretion and Cardiovascular Disease Mortality," *Journal of the American Medical Association* 306 (2011): 1083–87; and P. K. Whelton, "Urinary Sodium and Cardiovascular Disease Risk: Informing Guidelines for Sodium Consumption," *Journal of the American Medical Association* 306 (2011): 2262–64.

The meta-analysis mentioned is R. S. Taylor et al., "Reduced Dietary Salt for the Prevention of Cardiovascular Disease: A Meta-Analysis of Randomized Controlled Trials (Cochrane Review)," *American Journal of Hypertension* 24 (2011): 843–53. The editorial on it is M. H. Alderman, "The Cochrane Review of Sodium and Health," *American Journal of Hypertension* 24 (2011): 854–56. "It's Time to End the War on Salt" appeared in *Scientific American* on July 8, 2011. The notice that the Taylor meta-analysis was withdrawn is posted at the *Cochrane Database of Systematic Reviews* (2013): CD009217; the study that was removed from the meta-analysis was S. Paterna et al., "Normal-Sodium Diet Compared with Low-Sodium Diet in Compensated Congestive Heart Failure: Is Sodium an Old Enemy or a New Friend?" *Clinical Science* 114 (2008): 221–30. The discredited article from this research group is J. J. DiNicolantonio et al., "Low Sodium Versus Normal Sodium Diets in Systolic Heart Failure: Systematic Review and Meta-Analysis," *Heart* (2013), doi:10.1136/heartjnl-2012-302337. The entire topic of the duplicated and subsequently missing data is discussed at http://retractionwatch.com. The meta-analysis that excluded the suspect study is F. J. He and G. A. MacGregor, "Salt Reduction Lowers Cardiovascular Risk: Meta-Analysis of Outcome Trials," *Lancet* 378 (2011): 380–81.

The Institute of Medicine report on salt is *Sodium Intake in Populations: Assessment of the Evidence* (Washington, DC: National Academies Press, 2013), and the editorial about it is M. H. Alderman and H. W. Cohen, "The IOM Report Fails to Detect Evidence to Support Dietary Sodium Guidelines," *American Journal of Hypertension* 26 (2013): 1198–200.

The FDA's docket on salt is number FDA-2011-N-0400.

The story of how Congress blocked the publication of the guidelines on food marketing to children was described by Marion Nestle at http://www.foodpolitics.com on January 16, 2014.

The Sodium Reduction Strategy for Canada (July 2010) is available at http://www.hc-sc.gc.ca.

Christine Curtis's study on sodium changes is C. J. Curtis et al., "Change in Sodium Density in the U.S. Packaged Food Supply, 2009–2012." At this writing, the study is under review at a scientific journal. The study I used to estimate the impact of these changes on mortality in the United States is K. Bibbins-Domingo et al., "Projected Effect of Dietary Salt Reductions on Future Cardiovascular Disease," *New England Journal of Medicine* 362 (2010): 590–99.

Chapter 18: *"This is an attack on small business."*

Information about the ties between Coca-Cola and both the NAACP and the Hispanic Federation is in "In NAACP, Industry Gets Ally Against Soda Ban," *New York Times*, January 23, 2013.

Payments from the beverage companies to the city of Chicago are described in: "Beverage Giants Offer City $5 Million Prize to Avoid New Tax," *Chicago Sun-Times*, October 8, 2012; "Coca-Cola Gives $3M to City for Anti-Obesity, Diabetes Efforts," *Chicago Tribune*, November 12, 2012; and "Key Member of Rahm's Communications Team Joining Coca-Cola," *Chicago Sun-Times* July 29, 2013.

The legal cases mentioned are *Boreali v. Axelrod,* 71 N.Y.2d 1 (1987); *Metropolitan Board of Health v. Heister,* 37 N.Y. 661 (1868); *Paduano v. City of New York,* 257 N.Y.2d 531 (1965); and *Sorbonne Apartments Co. v. Board of Health of the City of New York,* 88 Misc. 2d 970; 390 N.Y.2d 358 (1976).

The portion cap legal case is *New York Statewide Coalition of Hispanic Chambers of Commerce v. New York City Department of Health,* 970 N.Y.2d 200 (2013).

The quote from the legal argument comes from "Fight over Bloomberg's Soda Ban Reaches Courtroom," *New York Times,* January 23, 2013 (original article no longer on *New York Times* website but available at www.newsdiffs.org).

Chapter 19: *"It keeps me up at night."*

The town of Haverstraw's experience with a tobacco display ban is recounted in L. E. Curry et al., "The Haverstraw Experience: The First Tobacco Product Display Ban in the United States," *American Journal of Public Health* 104 (2014): e9–e12.

The studies mentioned on the potential value of the law raising the sales age of tobacco to twenty-one are: J. DiFranza and M. Coleman, "Sources of Tobacco for Youths in Communities with Strong Enforcement of Youth Access Laws," *Tobacco Control* 10 (2001): 323–28; S. Ahmad, "Closing the Youth Access Gap: The Projected Health Benefits and Cost Savings of a National Policy to Raise the Legal Smoking Age to 21 in the United States," *Health Policy* 75 (2005): 74–84; A. Wagenaar and T. Toomey, "Effects of Minimum Drinking Age Laws: Review and Analysis of the Literature from 1960–2000," *Journal of Studies on Alcohol,* supp. 14 (2002): S206–S225. Data on smoking trends among the Needham high school students comes from the town's health department; comparison data for that region of Massachusetts is available in the "MetroWest Region High School Report 2012," available at http://www.mwhealth.org.

Transcripts from all New York City Council hearings are posted at http://council.nyc.gov.

The report in which the U.S. surgeon general concluded that smoking in movies causes youth to start smoking is *Preventing Tobacco Use Among Young Adults* (Atlanta: U.S. Department of Health and Human Services, CDC, 2012). The prospective study of children and movie exposure is L. Titus-Ernstoff et al., "Longitudinal Study of Viewing Smoking in Movies and Initiation of Smoking in Children," *Pediatrics* 121 (2008): 15–21.

The e-cigarette brands marketed by the big three tobacco companies (before a proposed merger of Reynolds America and Lorillard) were Blu (Lorillard), Vuse (R.J. Reynolds), and MarkTen (Altria, Philip Morris). For the invention of electronic cigarettes, see "A High-Tech Approach to Getting a Nicotine Fix," *Los Angeles Times*, April 25, 2009. Some of the business aspects are described in "Vapor Trails," *Business North Carolina*, March 2013, available at http://www .businessnc.com/articles/2013-03/vapor-trails-category.

The profile on Sean Parker is "Sean Parker: Agent of Disruption," *Forbes*, September 21, 2011.

Chapter 20: *"That is, ultimately, government's highest duty."*

Statistics on noncommunicable disease mortality globally are available in R. Lozano et al., "Global and Regional Mortality from 235 Causes of Death for 20 Age Groups in 1990 and 2010: A Systematic Analysis for the Global Burden of Disease Study 2010," *Lancet* 380 (2012): 2095–128, and at the website for the Institute for Health Metrics and Evaluation, http://www.healthdata.org. The UN secretary general's report *Prevention and Control of Non-Communicable Diseases* (A/66/83) is available at http://www.un.org/en/ga/ncdmeeting2011/documents .shtml.

Articles on the life expectancy gains in New York City include "Increased Life Expectancy in New York City: What Accounts for the Gains," *Epi Research Report*, Department of Health and Mental Hygiene (March 2013); T. Alcorn, "Redefining Public Health in New York City," *Lancet* 379 (2012): 2037–38; and S. H. Preston and I. T. Elo, "Anatomy of a Municipal Triumph: New York City's Upsurge in Life Expectancy," *Population and Development Review* 40 (2014): 1–29. The comparison of life expectancy gains in New York City to those of other major U.S. cities is based on data provided by the Institute for Health Metrics and Evaluation.

Data on smoking rates by year in both adults and high school students are available through the health department's EpiQuery tool at: https://a816 -healthpsi.nyc.gov/epiquery.

Data on on-screen smoking are available at http://www.cdc.gov/tobacco/ data_statistics/fact_sheets/youth_data/movies/index.htm.

The global antismoking work of Bloomberg Philanthropies is described in the organization's report "Accelerating the Worldwide Movement to Reduce Tobacco Use," Fall 2011, available at http://www.bloomberg.org. The status of global tobacco control is summarized in the *WHO Report on the Global Tobacco Epidemic, 2013*, available at http://www.who.int. The estimate of lives saved from global tobacco control comes from a model that was developed by David T. Levy and used for many other settings.

The estimate of the number of deaths attributable to unhealthy diet in America comes from the Institute of Health Metric and Evaluation's analysis, accessed with its GBD Compare tool at http://vizhub.healthdata.org/gbd-compare. The prevalence of obesity in America comes from C. L. Ogden et al., "Prevalence of Childhood and Adult Obesity in the United States, 2011–2012," *Journal of the American Medical Association* 311 (2014): 806–14.

In Seattle, calorie labeling in restaurants was not followed by reductions in the calorie content of food purchases six months later, but eighteen months later it was, as shown in J. W. Krieger et al., "Menu Labeling Regulations and Calories Purchased at Chain Restaurants," *American Journal of Preventive Medicine* 44 (2013): 595–604.

The increase in availability of fruits and vegetables in neighborhoods in which Green Carts were operating is described in the health department's *Epi Data Brief* no. 48, "Green Cart Evaluation, 2008–2011," August 2014.

The health department's food standards can be found at: http://www.nyc.gov/html/doh/html/living/agency-food-standards.shtml.

The FDA's final menu labeling rule is available at: http://www.fda.gov/Food/IngredientsPackagingLabeling/LabelingNutrition/ucm217762.htm.

Two randomized controlled trials on the effects of sugary drinks are J. C. de Ruyter et al., "A Trial of Sugar-Free or Sugar-Sweetened Beverages and Body Weight in Children," *New England Journal of Medicine* 367 (2012): 1397–406; and C. B. Ebbeling et al., "A Randomized Trial of Sugar-Sweetened Beverages and Adolescent Body Weight," *New England Journal of Medicine* 367 (2012): 1407–16.

The New York State court of appeals decision on the portion cap case is available at https://www.nycourts.gov/ctapps/Decisions/2014/Jun14/134opn14-Decision.pdf.

The global obesity epidemic is described in M. Ng et al., "Global, Regional, and National Prevalence of Overweight and Obesity in Children and Adults During 1980–2013; A Systematic Analysis for the Global Burden of Disease Study 2013," *Lancet* 384 (2014): 766–81. The Bloomberg foundation's involvement in the Mexican soda tax is briefly described at http://www.bloomberg.org/program/public-health/obesity-prevention. Comments on the impact of this tax on sugary drink sales are in "Mexico Soda Tax Dents Coke Bottler's Sales," *Wall Street Journal*, February 26, 2014. On the battles for the Berkeley soda tax initiative, see "How Michael Bloomberg Helped Pass Berkeley's Soda Tax," *Washington Post*, November 6, 2014.

Thanks

Thanks first to Michael Bloomberg, who could have spent his money and his political power on many things but chose to spend them helping New Yorkers live longer, healthier lives. If you ask me, that is what the mayoralty is for. And thanks to him for then giving a few hundred million dollars to prevent needless suffering in places like Bangladesh. I can think of no better way to use a fortune. Thanks to Tom Frieden for applying his greatest strength—his relentlessness—to save lives. And thanks to both men for entrusting New Yorkers' health to this untested professor from New Orleans.

The New York City Department of Health and Mental Hygiene is indeed a powerhouse of intelligence, creativity, and compassion. The staff members who spoke to me for this book are Sonia Angell, Mary Bassett, Anna Caffarelli, Eve Cagan, Louise Cohen, Geoff Cowley, Christina Chang, Kelly Christ, Christine Curtis, Blayne Cutler, Jeffrey Escoffier, Tom Frieden, Andy Goodman, Victoria Grimshaw, Daliah Heller, Susan Kansagra, Maura Kennelly, Beth Kilgore, Ashley Lederer, Wilfredo Lopez, Chris Manning, Elliott Marcus, Colin McCord, Tom Merrill, Sam Miller, Farzad Mostashari, Amanda Parsons, Anne Pearson, Sarah Perl, Andrew Rein, Lynn Silver, Kevin Schroth, Donna Shelley, Anne Sperling, Monica Sweeney, and Lorna Thorpe. Thanks to them and to the thousands of others in the department who quietly protect and promote the health of all New Yorkers. Beside those listed above, some of the many who helped me run the agency were Julie Friesen, Carolyn Greene, Adam Karpati, Dan Kass, Jian Liu, Marisa Raphael, Assunta Rozza, Jay Varma, and Patsy Yang. Thanks to those who, at various times, served as my chief of staff, helping translate my ideas into plans and keeping me out of trouble: Christina Chang, Kelly Christ, Emiko Otsubo, and for a short time, Jonathan Wangel.

Thanks to others who sat for interviews, including Jose Bandujo, Bob Brothers, Linda Gibbs, Peter Madonia, Christine Quinn, Alfred Sommer, and Howard Wolfson. My apologies to those who gave me wonderful stories and insights that I wasn't able to fit into this short book. Thanks to Frank Maselli not just for showing me how the electronic medical record works but also for connecting me to Chris Gallin and Sylvia Birnbaum (not her real name), and thanks to those two for letting me tell their stories.

Writing a book takes a long time. Thanks to Laurie Tisch and Rick Luftglass for supporting the Joan H. Tisch fellowship and to Jennifer Raab at Hunter College for letting me occupy it so that I had that time. Jonathan Fanton, Jack Rosenthal, Fay Rosenfeld, Laura Holbrooke, and the others at Roosevelt House at Hunter College helped me work. Special thanks to Judith Rodin, Peter Madonia, Pilar Palacio, and others at the Rockefeller Foundation for giving me three glorious weeks in Bellagio to think and write in a sea of creativity.

Tom Mayer at W. W. Norton made this book shorter and much better. Not many authors today are fortunate enough to get that kind of help. Katherine Fausset of Curtis Brown helped me think through the book and persuaded Tom Mayer that it was worth a try.

Index